THE
ALL-PRO
DIET

THE ALL-PRO DIET

LOSE FAT, BUILD MUSCLE, AND LIVE LIKE A CHAMPION

TONY GONZALEZ

WITH MITZI DULAN, RD

RODALE

© 2009 by Tony Gonzalez

Rodale books may be purchased for business or promotional use or for special sales. For information, please write to:
Special Markets Department, Rodale Inc., 733 Third Avenue, New York, NY 10017

Printed in the United States of America
Rodale Inc. makes every effort to use acid-free ∞, recycled paper ♻.

Photographs by Blaine Fisher/Getty Images

Book design by Christopher Rhoads

Library of Congress Cataloging-in-Publication Data

Gonzalez, Tony, 1976-
    The all-pro diet : lose fat, build muscle, and live like a champion / Tony Gonzalez with Mitzi Dulan.
        p.   cm.
    ISBN-13 978–1–60529–951–8 hardcover
    ISBN-10 1–60529–951–0 hardcover
    1. Athletes—Nutrition—United States.   2. Football players—Nutrition—United States.
    3. Gonzalez, Tony, 1976-   4. Physical fitness—Nutritional aspects.   I. Dulan, Mitzi.   II. Title.
TX361.A8G65   2009
613.2'024796—dc22   2009016872

Distributed to the trade by Macmillan

2 4 6 8 10 9 7 5 3 1   hardcover

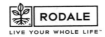

RODALE
LIVE YOUR WHOLE LIFE™

We inspire and enable people to improve their lives and the world around them

For more of our products visit **rodalestore.com** or call 800-848-4735

To my family, for all of your support throughout the years.
To my wife, October, for putting up with my being the food police.
—Tony

To Antoine, with much love and gratitude for all that you do.
—Mitzi

CONTENTS

Acknowledgments   ix

Introduction   xi

PART 1

THE ULTIMATE NUTRITION PACKAGE

CHAPTER 1. MY PLAN OF ACTION   3

CHAPTER 2. SEE THE GOALS   17

CHAPTER 3. THE 17 ALL-PRO DIET PRINCIPLES   38

CHAPTER 4. PREPARE FOR THE HIKE   61

CHAPTER 5. THE ALL-PRO DIET PLAN   77

CHAPTER 6. GETTING STARTED WITH THE ALL-PRO DIET MEAL PLAN   99

CHAPTER 7. ALL-PRO RECIPES   123

PART 2

THE ULTIMATE FITNESS PROGRAM: TONY G'S ALL-PRO WORKOUT

CHAPTER 8. EATING FOR PERFORMANCE   163

CHAPTER 9. PRIMED FOR PEAK PERFORMANCE   173

PART 3

THE ALL-PRO MINDSET FOR SUCCESS

CHAPTER 10. INTRODUCTION TO THE 8-POINT PLAN OF ATTACK   203

Appendix A. Know the Difference Between a Nutritionist and a Registered Dietitian   219

Appendix B. Statements from Authorities   221

Resource Guide   227

Index   231

ACKNOWLEDGMENTS

Thanks to all of you for buying this book, keeping an open mind, and taking a step in the right direction for your health.

Thanks to the random guy on the plane who recommended I read the book that started me on this nutrition journey.

Thanks to Dr. Colin Campbell for writing *The China Study*.

To my coauthor, Mitzi Dulan, thanks for your persistent effort and dedication to this book.

Thank you to the entire Rodale team. To Ed Claflin, thanks for your editorial magic. Thanks to Scott Ostler.

Thanks to Coach Vermeil, Coach Edwards, Jeff Hurd, Cedric Smith, and Jon Hinds.

Thank you to my attorney, Arash Khalili.

Last but not least, thanks to my entire family; you have blessed me with your encouragement, support, and unconditional love over the years. To my wife, October, and my amazing children, Nikko and Malia, you are the reason I want to live a long and healthy life.

—*Tony Gonzalez*

I'd first like to thank Tony Gonzalez for believing that we had an important message to share and giving me the opportunity to work with you on this project. You are an outstanding football player but an even better person.

To my husband, Antoine; an amazing father and husband who was always willing to pick up the slack during the many times I needed to work on the book. Thanks for allowing our home to be the official test kitchen for all of the recipes. To my wonderful daughters, Josie and Jasmine, thanks for making my life so much fun with your joyous spirits.

Thanks to all of my clients, friends, and colleagues who have provided encouragement throughout this journey, including: Kate Geagan, Felicia Stoler, Shelly Marie, Robin Plotkin, Cindy Heroux, Chris Mohr, Patti Puricelli, and Katie Hamm.

Thanks to all the wonderful people at Rodale including: Courtney Conroy, Julie Will, and Blanca Oliviery. Also, thank you Scott Ostler. Ed Claflin, thanks for all of your amazing editorial work.

My late mother, Lois, I am eternally grateful to you and dad, Galen, for all of your unconditional love. Mom, you were always so selfless. Thanks to my brother, Nick, who has always supported me and took me to my first Chiefs game when I was 16.

—*Mitzi Dulan*

INTRODUCTION

When I was in high school, I ate the kind of stuff that the average, unhealthy American kid loves to eat. Burgers with bacon and cheese. Deep-fried chicken wings. Shrimp drenched in butter. Steak—at least three times a week. The perfect breakfast was an egg and cheese omelet and white-bread toast slathered with butter and jam. After school, or whenever I got the chance, I'd head off to Burger King, McDonald's, or Taco Bell to chow down with the guys.

Sure, I was big into sports. I burned calories like nobody's business. But what I didn't know back then was where my diet was taking me. I was on a crash course, headed for the kind of future that just about every American kid faces these days—especially the kids who eat the way I did: a one-in-three chance of developing type 2 diabetes or prediabetes as an adult. A soaring risk of high blood pressure, putting me among the millions on the verge of heart attack or stroke. A big possibility that, if nothing changed, I would become one of those obese Americans dealing with all the consequences of insulin resistance and high cholesterol as well as high blood sugar and high triglycerides.

Of course, back then, I didn't pay much attention to what I was eating. Playing football was the center of my life—just as it had been ever since I was a little kid struggling to make my first Pop Warner team. But that was then, and this is now. After more than a decade on the big stage in the National Football League, I have a lot more appreciation for all the things the human body can do—and what it can't do.

What it can do, I've learned, is work hard, run fast, and be pushed to the limits of exhaustion. An athlete's body can put up with punishing workouts, muscle strains, bruises, sprains, and fractures. After a long season, it can repair a lot of damage that's been done and recover from innumerable hard hits and body blows.

But I've also learned what my body can't do. My liver and kidneys can't handle huge amounts of processed carbohydrates. My arteries can't deal with huge quantities of sticky plaque that interferes with blood flow. My nerves and brain cells have some minimum mineral requirements—and if those requirements aren't met, my energy and response times suffer the consequences. And all parts of my body—the parts I punish and damage and push to the max—need a constant supply of the right kind of nutrients to mend, preserve, heal, and prevent the onset of disease.

Right now, the biggest part of my life is football. But I'm not a kid in the Pop Warner league anymore, and I know a lot better than any kid can understand that there has to be life beyond football, too. That's why I don't eat the way I used to.

The fact is, I'm beginning to focus a lot of my time and energy on having a great life and success beyond my football career. I'm talking about staying healthy and fit for the long run.

Don't get me wrong: Nothing is as much fun as catching a football with the game hanging in the balance. The excitement of playing big-time football in front of huge crowds is awesome. I'm constantly pushing myself, and I'm never satisfied with last year's record or last week's performance on the field. But at the end of each NFL season, when I play my final game, I don't want to be facing a lifelong struggle with obesity and its many consequences. I've seen retired football players go that route. And thanks, but I'd prefer to avoid that kind of future.

My nutritionist, Mitzi Dulan, has worked wonders in getting NFL and MLB players to pay closer attention to health issues. I've already seen the impact of her advice on my own health, and I want to get the message out there. In fact, that's one of the reasons I decided to write this book. I have genuine concern for the health of NFL players. I'm not just a guy out to turn my own life around. I want to help you improve the quality of your life through my program, and I also want to share what I've learned with other guys in the NFL. My opinion is that a qualified sports nutritionist should focus on making sure the player is healthy and able to perform at a peak level through a proper diet plan. The NFL is changing, and the studies they are conducting, along with their greater emphasis on player health, reflect those changes. My goal is to help push for these changes by spreading the word about how to eat and what to eat for optimum health, mental clarity, and peak performance. Mitzi has told me that more than 75 percent of all NFL teams currently have sports dietitians working with their players. We know the name of the game is performance, but now I know that I don't have to sacrifice my health to perform at the top of my game. The reality is that I'm eating better and performing better on the football field as a result.

But I have another reason for writing this book, and that reason is you. With all I've learned recently about Americans' health and our nutritional problems—plus the input I've been getting from nutritionists—I've realized that a lot of us are dealing with health issues stemming from being overweight or obese. And our weight is directly related to our lifestyle, our diet, and the amount of exercise we get every day.

Although I call it the All-Pro Diet, you don't have to be a pro player to get the benefits of the kind of food and lifestyle choices that I recommend in this book. Women and men of all ages can benefit, and so can kids. This isn't just another diet book that promises you will lose X number of pounds in just a week or a month. What I'm proposing is a new *way* of eating—choosing food that tastes good and is good for you. Yes, it may be a big change, but it's not a change you have to make all at once. It will take some time. As I like to say, *slow down before you turn around.*

Often, when people "go on a diet," they have an all-or-nothing mentality. They start something and then stop. But the All-Pro Diet isn't something you try for 2 weeks, a month, or 7 months and then go back to your old habits. With this diet, eating is pleasurable, habits change over time, and after a while, you won't feel like you're being deprived of anything. You'll see—and feel—the benefits. And that's the greatest inspiration of all.

The changes I've made are for future health as well as current physical performance and well-being. I'm no longer that kid who stuffed himself with whatever food came his way. With luck and a little education, I've made the necessary changes in time to avoid the health problems that a kid like that inevitably faces. Yes, deep down inside, that kid is still there, wanting to hang out with his pals at the nearest burger joint. But I can look forward as well as back. And what I'm looking forward to is the opportunity to take the road to wellness.

If you care to join me on that road—and I hope you do—read on!

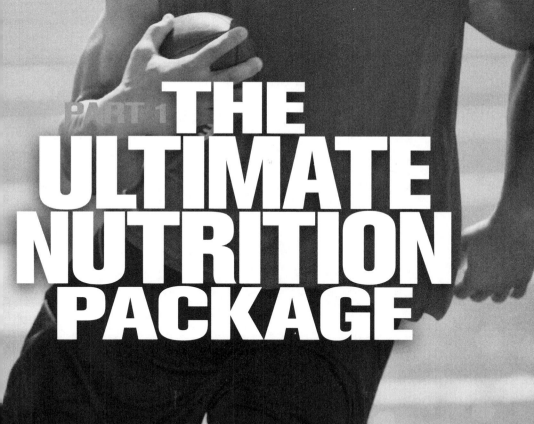

PART 1

THE ULTIMATE NUTRITION PACKAGE

CHAPTER 1

MY PLAN OF ACTION

"CHANGING YOUR DIET JUST MIGHT SAVE YOUR LIFE."

—Mitzi Dulan

In this book, I'm going to share a nutrition and lifestyle plan that will help you lose weight, gain muscle, and live a healthier life. I want to emphasize, first of all, that this isn't some gimmicky diet and exercise program that guarantees you'll lose X number of pounds per week or develop the kind of washboard abs that will earn you the Mr. Fitness award. But I can guarantee this: It's a plan that works for me.

It's true that you don't have quite as much at stake as I do. In all likelihood, your next year's employment contract does not depend on being strong, fit, and ready for the once-a-week thunder of an all-consuming NFL game. I'm willing to bet your Sunday afternoons during football season are considerably more relaxing than mine. You may not feel compelled, as I do, to jump rope a thousand times or bench-press a couple hundred pounds. But still, I'll bet there's one very important thing that you and I have in common. We like to feel good. We like to wake up with plenty of energy and feel invigorated rather than exhausted when we exercise. I'll bet you like the feeling of being fit as much as I do. And, yup, I'll bet you even love to *eat* as much as I do—but you hate the feeling of carrying around a lot of excess fat on your body.

So here's what we share (I'll bet): a healthy respect for feeling good.

Here's what we don't like (I'll bet again): feeling like a slug.

And here's what we really dread (my final bet): losing our health.

THE PLUSES FOR EVERYONE

What if I told you I could come up with a total plan that would help you have more endurance, better focus, and faster recovery? Wouldn't you be interested? Even if you're not a pro athlete, these are things all of us want. Here's what I mean:

More energy and endurance—You last longer when everyone else is getting tired.

Better focus—In the meeting room, in the classroom, at home, out on the field; wherever you are, you have greater ability to concentrate on what needs to be done. And that means you're not going to let other people down!

Faster recovery—The day after working out hard or playing a tough game, you come back feeling fresh and full of energy. The other guys may look at you like you're crazy, but you really have that kind of bounce-back capability. They're aching and hurting and moaning and, sure, you've got a few bumps and bruises, but you're ready to go again!

These were all the benefits I started to experience when I switched to the All-Pro Diet that I describe in this book. It all adds up to better performance. For a professional athlete, having more endurance, better focus, and faster recovery means being able to work harder and play better than ever before. And that means a longer career. For a young athlete, it means making the A team instead of the B team, which might mean getting the athletic scholarship instead of someone else. However, it is in no way all about money—more importantly, this is about your lifelong health. For everyone else, more endurance, better focus, and faster recovery means not letting teammates or colleagues down, staying in the game, and coming in fresh and full of energy no matter what the activity. Who *wouldn't* make this choice? It's a no-brainer.

This lifestyle program can make the biggest difference in the world. It's more than a nutrition and exercise program. It's also the mental work that you do to make yourself better. And that's what it's all about. Focus on getting better—all the time—and no matter how you look at it, you're going to come closer to achieving your dreams. It's really worth it!

THE HEALTH DIMENSION

What are the benefits of switching over to a different kind of diet?

I can only speak for myself, of course. But I've also done some reading on the subject—enough to sound a few alarms about the way most of us eat today. And by "most of us," I'm not talking just about football players.

The wake-up call regarding my own health came in the form of two unrelated crises. My first big scare came when I was diagnosed with Bell's palsy, a form of temporary facial paralysis resulting from damage or trauma to one of two facial nerves. It's not a condition that can be immediately diagnosed, and before the doctors figured out what it was, they told me I might have had a stroke, a brain aneurysm, or meningitis. I was rushed to the hospital, where they immediately performed a CAT scan. During that long ride and the examination that followed, I had the opportunity to do some very serious soul-searching about the direction my life was taking.

I was lucky! When the tests showed I had Bell's palsy, the doctors assured me that there was about a four-in-five chance that I would recover fully. If all went well, my initial symptoms—the numbness and sagging features—would right themselves without any serious aftereffects. Many people with Bell's palsy get over it without ever having a recurrence. As it turned out, an acupuncture treatment was extremely helpful to me, and the paralysis went away in 2 weeks.

But another health scare lay ahead. Just before the 2007–2008 football season, I went for my annual preseason physical in Kansas City. As usual, I had a blood test at the hospital. As I was leaving town to head back home to California, I got a call from the team trainer. He told me my white blood cell count was dangerously low. I had to return immediately for another blood test.

> **"GIVEN WHAT I DO FOR A LIVING, MY BODY IS MY TEMPLE—AND YOU NEED TO PUT THE RIGHT THINGS IN YOUR BODY. IF YOU ARE NOT EATING THE RIGHT THINGS OR GETTING THE PROPER AMOUNT OF REST, YOU WON'T BE PRODUCTIVE."**
>
> —Tony Richardson, 15-Year NFL Veteran

Back in Kansas City, as I gave blood for the second time, I was told by the doctor that unless the first test was wrong, my football career was over. I was facing a serious medical situation. Again, I suffered through a prolonged waiting period when, it seemed, my whole life hung in the balance. Would I ever walk out on the gridiron again? Was my career really over? Suddenly, I was seeing my life from a completely different perspective—

GOOD EATING—IT'S INFECTIOUS!

"NFL players reflect similar eating challenges that many other men face and their nutrition concerns are as varied and individual as the number of players on a team. Knowing how much to eat, when to eat, and what to eat are questions many players ask. Figuring out how to prepare or purchase the foods that will both fuel and nourish them is an ongoing task. One of the goals of the team nutritionist is to help the athlete find what works best for that individual in considering training and recovery demands, food preferences, health history, and ideology while keeping lifestyle and performance goals in mind."

—Heidi Skolnik, MS, CDN, FACSM, Team Nutritionist for the New York Giants from the point of view of someone who might have only months to live. It was a shock. After the doctor called me, I can remember driving in my car with tears running down my face.

To my incredible relief, the second test came back normal. It turned out the lab had confused my blood test results with those of another patient. It was a terrible error, and I can't imagine what it was like for the person who had to be told the bad news. But for the moment, I had dodged the bullet.

Though relieved, I still felt sobered by these experiences. Each time, I was reminded just how important my good health is to me and how much I take it for granted. Yet, at the same time, I was reading books like *The China Study* by T. Colin Campbell, an author who offered clear statistical and epidemiological evidence that my diet was a train wreck just waiting to happen.

The convincing proof was mounting every day. I wasn't the only one on a diet that was steering me toward health disaster. Millions of other Americans were on the same track. And the American culinary landscape—from the fast-food dens of double-sized drinks and triple-sized burgers to the mountains of highly advertised packaged and processed food products filling the shelves of enormous supermarkets—had caused the staggering obesity of an overfed yet undernourished population. I realized that many of us are, quite literally, the walking wounded, not because of what we've suffered in war and destitution but because of the way we've filled our plates and fed our hunger.

MEET MS. DULAN

It's time to introduce one of my favorite people, a friend and expert dietitian who has been instrumental in developing the incredible nutrition plan that I call the All-Pro Diet. Mitzi Dulan, RD, is one of the top nutritionists working in the NFL.

Mitzi and I first discussed my nutrition in 2004, when I consulted with her about my eating habits. This marked the point where I thought I was ready to take action.

For more than 10 years, Mitzi had been doing nutritional consulting with professional athletes from all major sports. She worked for the Golden State Warriors and San Jose Sharks before taking over as the team nutritionist for the Kansas City Chiefs and the Kansas City Royals. Not only a registered dietitian with the highest certification in sports nutrition, Mitzi is also a board-certified specialist in sports dietetics (CSSD), a position held by fewer than 300 nutritionists in the United States.

To tell the truth, when I first talked to Mitzi in 2004, I wasn't really ready to take her advice seriously. But a few years later—and after my health scares—I again sought out her opinion and advice about my diet. That was May 2007. It was around that time that I began doing a lot more reading. Mitzi encouraged me to learn the facts—and once I did, I became even more eager for change.

Just to give you some background on my state of mind at the time: I was at a stage in my career when I was realizing the need to be proactive about changing my nutrition plan. My old gobble-up-the-fat and wolf-down-the-calories lifestyle just wasn't doing it for me anymore. All around me, people were talking about the long-term damage of obesity. Here I was, a professional athlete relying on my body to perform, but I had hardly any understanding of what my body needed to perform at its best. I was reading about nutritional studies comparing the long-term health of people in different cultures, and I was hearing about the epidemic-proportion outbreak of type 2 diabetes among young people in the United States. Yet I was barely paying attention to the damage or the benefit of my own nutritional plan. In fact, I didn't have a plan. That began to seem more than foolish: It was downright irresponsible.

Given my greater receptivity to Mitzi's advice in 2007 compared to our first meeting, the question now was not whether I would begin to make changes, but how and when. I knew I needed guidance. And that's what Mitzi provided.

It didn't take Mitzi long to see that she'd be working with a guy who had once been addicted to junk food. In fact, she knew that already from our earlier meeting in 2004, when she suggested I decrease my cheese intake and cook more meals at home. I love cheese. My weakness was anything with cheese in it. And me, cook? Like most of the NFL players Mitzi works with, I was always eating out. I'd go to a restaurant, order anything that looked good—the more food, the better—and clean my plate. Pizza, steak, and hamburgers were the core staples of my diet. To Mitzi this was par for the course. When guys weigh an eighth of a ton or so, they tend to eat heartily. Sure, there's the challenge of turning that fodder into some kind of useful muscle, but that's what we do. Take heaps of calories, turn them into energy, and use

MITZI ADVISES . . .

The drastic changes Tony has made in his diet are remarkable. The fact that he has been able to experience a very noticeable difference in his energy level, recovery, and ultimately his performance by changing his diet should be a wake-up call for anyone. And I do mean anyone. If you are a stay-at-home mom and still trying to lose your baby weight, this diet will help you do it. I have two young daughters. I used the principles outlined in the All-Pro Diet to lose 20 pounds and get back to what I weighed when I started college. (Mind you, this was before I gained the freshman 20!) With this program, I reached that goal—and I've never looked back. So I have personal experience as well as a strong conviction that it works. Plus, I've seen how well it works for other people.

The best thing about my job is getting to help people improve their health and change their lives. It's very rewarding to see people benefit from those changes. Tony feels better now than at any other point in his career. The All-Pro Diet is one that I'd recommend to anyone trying to achieve peak performance levels—whether in a conference room, at home, or on a football field—while at the same time improving your health.

every last joule of that energy to get into the end zone. What's wrong with that?

There was nothing particularly wrong, as Mitzi patiently began to explain. But . . . what if it were possible to stoke the fire with the kind of fuel that burned more steadily and lasted longer? What if I loaded the furnace with the kind of calories that would more easily turn into muscle fiber? What if I started to use the kind of fuel that would keep the engine well-tuned instead of clogging my arteries, attacking my liver, and making my pancreas work overtime? I was still living in the days of leaded, polluting gasoline when there was high-octane premium all around me.

A Consensus of Nutritionists

The days of sports nutritionists standing on the sidelines, waiting to be called in to give occasional advice, are rapidly vanishing. Today, there's ever-increasing awareness on the part of owners, coaches, teams, and players that performance is directly related to health. With mounting evidence that the classic football player's diet affects Sunday afternoon performance and has direct long-term health consequences, nutritionists have moved to the forefront.

A shining example of this new development is Leslie Bonci, MPH, RD, a team sports dietitian for the Pittsburgh Steelers and the University of Pittsburgh Department of Athletics.

"I prioritize nutrition for the Pittsburgh Steelers based on the following three goals: to optimize performance, safeguard health, and promote career longevity," says Leslie. "Although the players are incredibly talented, they don't always get an A+ in eating healthy. Some players have health baggage such as elevated lipids, gout, or hypertension; modifying their diet still needs to be accomplished with an emphasis on sports nutrition, not a clinical or disease-management perspective. Tweaking food choices and eating habits can provide the offense for strong sports performance and the defense against future health problems."

During our first sessions together, Mitzi listened to some of the changes I was already making to my diet and provided some recommendations. First step: Increase my protein. Second step: Avoid highly processed soy foods, because in my attempt to eat a more plant-based diet, I was eating imitation meats loaded with sodium and other unhealthy ingredients. Third step: Drink a recovery beverage every day after practice.

When I started to follow Mitzi's nutrition guidelines, I felt the impact almost immediately. Within 2 to 3 weeks, I was actually feeling positive change in my energy, my stamina, and my reaction time. Granted, I'm someone who pays a lot of attention to what's going on in his body. I have to. But this wasn't just hyperawareness. It was the difference between waking up every morning with the blahs versus waking up feeling like I couldn't wait to go outside and get something *done.*

It was interesting. And the more I got into it, the more I began to realize that there was some good science behind Mitzi's recommendations. Once I got into the early stages of my new diet, I started asking her more questions and came to appreciate how much good information she had to offer.

As for Mitzi, having worked with professional athletes for more than 10 years, she was very good at sizing up an individual to see where he was "at"—from a nutritional standpoint—and how far he was willing to go. Some guys, I know, would be pretty tough to change. They're doing most of their fine dining at fast-food chains. They're winding up their workouts with little snacks such as four cookies the size of saucers. With those guys, Mitzi says, she starts with small steps. It is the only way to get them to where they ultimately need to be. She has to use the "just-a-little-bit-every-day" principle with them. Hey, you don't change the lifestyle of a 345-pound guard overnight. But Mitzi helps them see that they can do it if they just work hard 1 day at a time. Amazing things can happen. In fact, Mitzi preaches that compound effort creates big results. Even with *very* big linemen.

> **"ACHIEVEMENT IS LARGELY THE PRODUCT OF STEADILY RAISING ONE'S LEVELS OF ASPIRATION . . . AND EXPECTATION."**
>
> **—Jack Nicklaus, Professional Golfer**

By May 2007, I was ready to make any changes that would help me perform better and eat healthier. I approached the new diet the same way I approach football. If there was anything I could possibly do to improve, I wanted to try it. I was curious about the science behind nutrition, and every piece of new information was a valuable nugget. Before long, I found myself making mental notes of every single piece of advice that Mitzi had to offer. She answered all my questions to the best of her knowledge, gave me books to read, and whenever I asked, offered suggestions about things I could do to improve.

ARE YOU CONCERNED?

According to the latest statistics, about two-thirds of American adults are overweight or obese. In the past, more people were overweight than obese, but recently the numbers swapped, and now there are more obese Americans at 34 percent (over 72 million Americans) versus 32.7 percent who are overweight. (A whopping 6 percent are severely obese.) As you've probably realized from reading the headlines, children and adolescents are headed in the same direction, with an estimated 32 percent classified as overweight or obese. Childhood obesity has tripled in the past 20 years.

Not surprisingly, there is an alarming surge in the number of people with diseases that are closely related to, or directly caused by, being overweight or obese. Nearly 24 million adults have diabetes. About 50 percent of those with diabetes are between 20 and 60 years of age.

Many NFL players, unfortunately, suffer from all kinds of health conditions that are closely related to obesity. This is something that concerns me a lot. (As I mentioned earlier, it's one of my reasons for writing this book.) In a study conducted by Mayo Clinic physicians, of 223 retired

NFL players, researchers found that 82 percent of the players under the age of 50 already had some narrowing and blockages in their arteries. In addition to heart disease, it has been found that retired players often have significant problems with sleep apnea, depression, pain, obesity, high blood pressure, and diabetes.

As expected, men with these conditions are more likely to die prematurely. According to a study by Scripps Howard News Service of 3,850 professional athletes, heavy NFL players are twice as likely to die before age 50 as baseball players (who on average weigh much less). Among NFL players who die before age 50, frequent causes were found to be coronary disease, stroke, and cancer—again, the very conditions that are often associated with being overweight.

Many players have a family history of heart disease, hypertension, diabetes, and obesity even before they get into pro football. And of course weight gain is encouraged in the NFL. (The 300-pound football player was once rare, but now it's within the normal weight range for many offensive and defensive linemen.) In recent years, the NFL has made some progress in evaluating the health of current players. I think they need to continue to do more in order to assess the health risks of players, focus on identifying players with metabolic syndrome, and work to reduce their risk factors.

The health problems of retired NFL players are beginning to gain an increasing amount of media attention. But ultimately it's still up to each individual to take personal responsibility for his own diet and exercise program that will help prevent obesity and the health problems associated with it.

KNOW YOUR NUMBERS: DO YOU HAVE METABOLIC SYNDROME?

Are you one of the estimated 57 million Americans who have metabolic syndrome or prediabetes? Metabolic syndrome, also known as syndrome X, is characterized by a cluster of conditions known to increase the risk of both coronary heart disease and type 2 diabetes. It often starts with insulin resistance, which is when muscle, liver, and fat cells are insensitive to insulin. The insulin can no longer help take the glucose out of the blood and into the cell for use as energy, so the glucose stays in the blood and elevates the blood sugar level. The pancreas will continue to excrete insulin in an effort to bring the blood sugar down, but eventually it gets tired out.

Metabolic syndrome often goes undiagnosed because it is overlooked. If every NFL team were to look for and report the number of players who actually fall into the diagnosis of metabolic syndrome, my guess is that it would be a large number of guys. Many doctors don't look at the combination of conditions and truly recognize the significant associated cardiovascular risks. So when players see on lab results that they are not within normal limits, it should definitely be a kick in the butt for them to work hard to improve their numbers.

How do you find out if you have it? First, ask your doctor for a blood test to check your triglycerides, high-density lipoprotein (HDL), and fasting blood glucose. I even recommend a more advanced lipid test called a vertical auto profile (VAP) test, which is a very comprehensive cholesterol test measuring 15 different blood cholesterol components. Many insurance companies do not cover it, and it might cost about $100, but it would be worth the expense if it helps save your life! It was named one of the "five tests worth paying for" by the *Wall Street Journal*.

If you have three or more of the following five conditions, you have metabolic syndrome.

Condition	Indicator
Abdominal obesity (elevated waist circumference)	Men—Equal to or greater than 40 inches Women—Equal to or greater than 35 inches
Elevated triglycerides	Equal to or greater than 150 mg/dL
Reduced HDL ("good" cholesterol)	Men—less than 40 mg/dL Women—less than 50 mg/dL
Elevated blood pressure	Equal to or greater than 130/85 mmHg
Elevated fasting blood glucose	Equal to or greater than 100 mg/dL

Know Your Numbers

Date_____

My triglycerides_____

My HDL_____

My fasting blood glucose_____

My blood pressure_____

If you know someone with diabetes, he or she might have told you that it's under control. And it may be—with careful, regular monitoring and steady doses of medication. But its complications are not always under control, because there are so many, and they affect so many parts of the body. Three-quarters of adults with self-reported diabetes have high blood pressure, a leading risk factor for heart disease and stroke. (In a recent year, heart disease was noted on 68 percent of diabetes-related death certificates among people age 65 and older, while stroke was noted as the cause in 16 percent of cases.) Other closely related complications of diabetes include blindness, kidney disease, and nervous system diseases.

You can see why alarm bells should be going off. Most of us would assume that being overweight or obese is not the same as being told you've just had a stroke or been diagnosed with cancer. But that's where we're deluding ourselves. Obesity is the second leading cause of preventable death in the United States.

The word *preventable* means just that. When you swerve your car to avoid hitting a tree, that's a case in which death has been prevented. When you step back from a moving train, it's because you know a disaster is preventable—and you take steps to prevent it. Well, as it turns out, choosing better foods is the same as swerving to avoid the tree or stepping away from the speeding train. And we can make that choice easily, with the amazing range of foods that are available to us.

The 57 million Americans currently estimated to have metabolic syndrome are standing way too close to the tracks. And many, I'm afraid, aren't even aware that they have a largely preventable disease.

Of course, we all know that genetics play some role in how our bodies are shaped and how food is metabolized (the process of turning calories of food into calories of energy). I guess I'm a pretty good example of what can't be changed. I don't exactly have a delicate frame. But even so, I'm aware of my choices—and becoming more aware every day. While excess weight has never really been an issue for me because I exercise so frequently, I can foresee the day—given my genetics—when I could easily gain a lot of weight. That's why I want to make important choices now and eat the kinds of foods that help support my body's working parts. With the All-Pro Diet, I get to eat a lot of nutrient-rich foods that provide nourishment (for my energy needs) without a lot of empty calories (that don't provide much nutritional value or disease-fighting benefits).

The difference?

It's just a matter of paying attention.

CHAPTER 2

SEE THE GOALS

"WHAT WOULD HAPPEN IF WE WERE TO START THINKING ABOUT FOOD AS LESS OF A THING AND MORE OF A RELATIONSHIP?"

—Michael Pollan

I've mentioned a book by T. Colin Campbell called *The China Study* that initially had a big impact on my thinking. Campbell advocates a diet that consists largely of fruits, vegetables, nuts, whole grains, and legumes. In addition to avoiding all dairy, we should also ban meat, poultry, and eggs. It's essentially a book that recommends a plant-based, whole foods diet.

As I read Campbell's work, I found many of his arguments convincing. At first, I tried to be totally committed to it. In fact, there were a number of stories in the media about how I'd become a vegan, and those stories follow me around to this day even though I'm not one.

There are good reasons why I didn't stick with a fully plant-based diet. I found that when I totally cut out all animal products including meat and dairy, my performance was affected—and not in a positive way. Much of that was likely caused by the lack of protein in my diet. About the time I started on a plant-based diet, I recall former right guard for the Chiefs, John Wellbourn, shaking his head and saying, "Hey, China Study, you ain't gonna be able to move those 300-pound defensive ends!"

Maybe he had a point. I was fresh off my eighth consecutive Pro Bowl appearance, but past records don't impress anyone. In the NFL, you earn or lose respect on every play. I've seen players go from dominating to dominated in a heartbeat.

When another teammate, Jason Dunn, a former tight end for the Chiefs, challenged me on my new diet, I told him, "We'll see if it works. If I go out there and get my ass kicked the first few weeks, I'll go back to eating steak and french fries."

Of course, I didn't want to do that. I wanted to prove that I could eat a healthful diet and, at the same time, play my best. But on the other hand, this was no time to take a gamble. I had just signed a 5-year

MITZI ADVISES . . .

When Tony started his diet, he asked me to list the foods that, in my opinion, were the 10 *worst* and those that were the 10 *best*. Here's my selection.

THE TOP 10 WORST FOODS (IN NO PARTICULAR ORDER)

- Bacon
- Cheese sauce from a jar
- Commercially baked cookies and cakes
- Double cheeseburgers
- Doughnuts
- French fries
- Fruit juice and fruit drinks
- Potato chips
- Soda
- Whipped topping

THE TOP 10 BEST FOODS (IN NO PARTICULAR ORDER)

- Blueberries
- Broccoli
- Legumes
- Oats
- Oranges
- Spinach
- Sweet potatoes
- Tomatoes
- Walnuts
- Wild salmon

contract extension, making me the highest-paid tight end ever, and I wanted to prove that I was worthy of that honor. So—was this new diet a mistake?

My stomach was bothering me. My face was breaking out like a teenager's. Switching to a diet so high in fiber so quickly gave me some gastrointestinal issues (if you know what I mean). Let's just say constipation was no longer an issue.

Maybe, after about 20 years of hard football, my body was breaking down. But there was some good news, too. I found I was no longer bothered as much by an old foot injury. Doctors had told me that my foot was never going to get better, that I'd just have to learn to deal with the chronic pain. And I do mean pain! Heck, I would have changed my diet for that sole reason had I known it might have helped my foot like it did. There's no scientific evidence, but I do know that my foot doesn't hurt nearly as much as it did before my diet change.

I hit the weight room and I was shocked. Normally I do sets with 130-pound weights, about six reps, but now I was struggling with the 100-pound weights. No arguing with the facts: I was way weaker!

This new diet wasn't working. I was thinking, "I cannot play like this." But I also knew I couldn't go back to my old diet, eating junk.

I just wasn't feeling good. And as I talked it over with Mitzi, I realized why. Campbell suggests protein is the cause of many health issues. In fact, he recommends a fairly low protein intake. That might work for some people, but a professional football player can definitely not get away with a low-protein diet.

So what was the best alternative?

Mitzi and I decided that my own diet plan would be based on some of Campbell's basic principles but modified to suit my needs as a professional athlete and in coordination with Mitzi's extensive knowledge of sports nutrition. The All-Pro Diet, as it has evolved, also emphasizes fruits, vegetables, legumes, whole grains, nuts, and fish. In addition, however, I include free-range poultry, eggs, and sometimes a little cheese. And in my own diet I eat a very small amount of grass-finished red meat, less than 18 ounces a month.

ON THE TRACK TO GOOD HEALTH

What began as a modest, step-by-step program to get me eating healthier evolved into a total nutrition program, the All-Pro Diet that I'm presenting in this book.

Originally, this program was designed just for me. It was meant to rescue me from the kind of long-term damage that I was bound to suffer if I continued eating the way I had been. It was designed to help me maintain top performance. That was the goal of it all—to help me fine-tune the muscles I needed to play my best, while minimizing the fat. (To an active guy like me, every extra ounce of fat is dead weight!) If all went well, the All-Pro Diet would prolong my career and help me get the most out of every moment in the training room and on the playing field.

What I've realized, however, is that this isn't a nutritional program exclusively for me. The sound nutritional, peak-performance advice from Mitzi that was incorporated into the All-Pro Diet applies to everyone. Never mind whether you want to score X number of touchdowns or rack up 1,000 yards in a season. *I* like that kind of stuff, but you? Maybe you want to enjoy a brisk walk on a summer day without getting winded, or you want more energy when you're raking leaves or shoveling snow. Maybe you have a golf or tennis game you want to improve. Maybe you want to look in the mirror and really like what you see. Maybe you want to go to bed at night without feeling like you've just used your belly as a dump truck, or you like starting your workday with a lot of energy.

Can the All-Pro Diet really help you achieve those goals? *Any* of them? *All* of them?

Here's my advice: Try it!

> **"GET EXCITED AND ENTHUSIASTIC ABOUT YOUR OWN DREAM.
> THIS EXCITEMENT IS LIKE A FOREST FIRE—YOU CAN SMELL IT, TASTE IT,
> AND SEE IT FROM A MILE AWAY."**
>
> —Denis Waitley, Author, Keynote Speaker, and Productivity Expert

GETTING THERE

What Mitzi and I devised is not a fad diet. We don't want you to go on it, then off it, which is the way that most diet plans work. We are not asking you to count calories or to embrace any extreme diet plans. The goal is for you to stop eating foods that have empty calories and are high in sugar, bad fats, and artificial ingredients. We will also ask you to cut back on your animal-product consumption and eat more plant-based foods. These are simple steps.

How long will it take before the All-Pro Diet becomes second nature to you? It took me about 6 months before I was following most of the guidelines in this book. I started changing my diet in the off-season, but I had to make adjustments as I got into the groove of the football season. In particular, it took some time to tweak different protein sources. In fact, I am still always working to improve my diet. During the past two seasons, Mitzi and I got into the habit of having lunch every Wednesday. I would use this time to ask her nutrition questions, and she would share a lot of information. In the days afterward, I'd make some of the adjustments we discussed, trying out new foods, adding ever more variety to my repertoire of meals and snacks.

When we started the All-Pro Diet, there was no comprehensive recipe list like the one you'll find on pages 124–160. It just grew and grew, as I became more adventurous in my eating and developed a taste for a greater variety of foods and flavors than I'd ever encountered before. Today, it amazes me to look back and realize how much of my diet had been made up of the old American standbys—whole-milk products, steak, cheeseburgers, french fries, spaghetti, pizza, and so on. It was as if I'd just blocked out all other foods from around the world. "Have you ever tried . . . ?" Mitzi would ask, naming a grain, fruit, or vegetable that can be found in just about any supermarket. Time and again, I had to shake my head—no, never have. And within a day or two, Mitzi would have a new recipe for me, featuring some delicious concoction incorporating flavors, textures, and spices that I'd never tasted.

THE TOP SEVEN WEIGHT-LOSS TIPS
FOR THE ARMCHAIR QUARTERBACK

On the All-Pro Diet, you'll automatically start to lose weight and—as long as you stick with Phase II, which we'll discuss in a moment—you'll keep the weight off. But what happens when you and the guys are sitting around on a Sunday afternoon watching football? Obviously, I don't want to discourage you from doing that. Go ahead and enjoy it. But while you're in that armchair enjoying the game, there may be a lot of food in the room that doesn't belong in your stomach—especially if you're trying to lose weight. Here are some armchair strategies that I strongly recommend:

1. Set out plenty of fresh fruit to snack on.

2. Go for grilled chicken or fish instead of burgers or ribs.

3. Pass on the soda and fruit juice.

4. Make some delicious Guacamole (see the recipe on page 157) instead of junk food and enjoy the healthy fats and nearly 20 beneficial nutrients. Serve with whole wheat crackers or multigrain tortilla chips.

5. If you want a beer, go ahead—have one or two. *Just* one or two. (You want to limit alcohol consumption to five drinks per week.)

6. Those high-fat potato chips, cookies, and cheese spreads? Pretend they don't exist.

7. Do your pushups and ab moves during commercials.

Before long, it dawned on me that my eating habits had turned into just that—*habits*. I'd been in a groove where I wasn't even paying attention to the many things that make eating such a pleasure. I'd been stuffing myself to capacity. But where was the pleasure in that? I wanted to taste my food again—to really savor my meals and enjoy the preparation as well as the consumption. Gradually, step-by-step, lesson by lesson, Wednesday lunch by Wednesday lunch, the pleasure of eating came into my life.

THE CHANGE BEGINS . . . AND NEVER ENDS

As with all her clients, Mitzi recommended that I base my diet on whole grains, fruits, and vegetables—and, from here on out, to avoid processed foods as much as possible. Later on, when she suggested certain foods like grass-fed meats and free-range poultry, we actually went out to visit the farms together near Kansas City. During the off-season, I go to a local farmers' market in California every Sunday. I love it! It is great to meet the farmers who are growing your food. There is something very special about the face-to-face contact. Seeing where these animals were raised helped me understand and appreciate where my daily food was coming from.

In discovering that nutrition is a science, I also learned that we are accumulating new information regarding it almost every day. Mitzi's special talent was in figuring out what works for everyone, from the pro athlete to the soccer mom. In fact, I learned, her own family eats just the kinds of food that Mitzi advocates. She always includes some plant-based meals in the family diet. (In fact, the Black Bean Soup recipe on page 137 is one of her family's favorites.) And like other mothers, she tries to minimize her family's exposure to antibiotics, hormones, and pesticides by choosing organic foods whenever possible, and she recommends that her clients do the same.

MITZI ADVISES . . .

For Tony—and for anyone else going for a highly nutritious diet—I recommend that you buy fruits and vegetables locally whenever possible. Every Saturday, I take my kids with me to pick up my two sacks of food from a local CSA (Community Supported Agriculture) group. It is a great way to support the local farmers and get fresh produce, poultry, meat, and dairy. My daughters always look forward to picking up the food from the farmers. Getting a weekly CSA box also helps you try new foods and eat a wider variety since they put specific seasonal items in your bags. If you prefer a different food, you are usually allowed to trade. Some of the recipes in this book were inspired by the foods that I got from my CSA, including the Napa Cabbage White Bean Soup (recipe on page 138).

In his book *In Defense of Food*, Michael Pollan says, "Cooking is one of the most important health consequences of buying food from local farmers." When you meet the farmers, you can also talk to them about how they grow their food and how they control pests. Buying farm-grown produce that's raised without pesticides is not only good for the environment; there's a growing body of evidence that it's good for your health as well. Research out of the University of California, Davis, for instance, suggests that organically grown fruits and vegetables contain higher amounts of vitamin C than ones raised with chemical fertilizers, sprayed with chemical pesticides, and mass harvested at the earliest possible moment. Even if the nutritional quality is the same, you can argue that organic foods contain fewer pesticides, which is a good thing.

THE POWER OF THIS DIET

As for the benefits, I'd like to share a few personal observations that have proven to me the effectiveness of the All-Pro Diet in building a better physique and enhancing sports performance. And I will outline what some of those benefits may be for you.

For one thing, this diet has affected my powers of recovery. Here's how I know: In my sixth season, I broke a bone in my left foot. It was a small bone, and I kept putting off surgery, playing that way for a full year.

Finally, I had it repaired, but afterward my foot still didn't seem to heal properly. It was incredibly sore. I was in a lot of pain. I started to limp, and because I kept trying to take pressure off the foot, that snowballed into other physical problems. What a mess!

When the team physician took a look at the foot, he told me it should have been healing. And maybe it was, but measured from a level-of-pain perspective, it didn't feel like it.

That was a crucial point in my career. The pain was so intense that I thought I might have to retire. On my key practice days (Wednesdays and Thursdays), I could run only about 12 plays before I would have to stop because my foot was feeling so bad. The team physician told me there was nothing else he could do, that I was suffering from an arthritic condition that didn't respond to treatment.

It was right about then that I switched over to the All-Pro Diet. (I should emphasize that nothing else in my routine changed at all.) And then something remarkable happened. The pain started going away almost immediately. Today, I'm able to practice the way I could before the injury. These days, I feel so strong that I can run 30 plays in practice.

Could my recovery be attributed entirely to a change in diet? I don't know for sure, but I can't account for it otherwise. And since I've stayed on the diet, my foot feels a whole heck of a lot better than before.

What I do know for certain is that the change in my diet has made me a better football player. Throughout my career, I've been very alert to signs of improvement in my ability as an athlete, and when I find

What's Your Health Profile?

Getting regular physicals is part of the routine in the NFL, and it's a good idea for everyone else, too. Always check with your physician when starting a new diet plan to make sure that any changes won't impact your overall health.

something that makes a significant difference, I stick with it. The results of staying with this diet are incontrovertible. I can see my improvement as well as feel the difference every day. This diet has really helped me improve my speed, my ability to shake off tackles, recover more quickly after games and workout sessions, and just feel better and healthier every day.

I'm not surprised that many of the other players on my team, having seen the results of my new diet, are asking me about it. The results have been reflected in my performance—and it's very hard to argue with my success. I caught 99 passes in 2007 and 96 in 2008. Following the diet change, I took the lead in the most touchdowns, most receptions, and most receiving yards for a tight end. I was lifting strong and bouncing back from heavy-duty workouts while the other players were sore and fatigued. By the end of the season, I noticed the guys were trying to eat healthier. They knew my All-Pro Diet was paying dividends.

WHAT DOES THE DIET DO FOR YOU?

As a nutritionist who works with a lot of high-performance athletes, Mitzi is in a good position to provide some perspective on these changes that have had such a big personal impact. She points out that my constant drive to improve my performance—something I've had ever since I was a kid—has been an asset when it comes to searching for ways to improve. By the age of 19, I was a big reader of Tony Robbins's books, and right there, I became very committed to setting goals. Once I realized how the All-Pro Diet was having such a positive impact on my performance, there was no turning back. My goal was to go with this new plan and explore it in every way possible to get maximum results. As Mitzi points out, I've got pretty good self-awareness when it comes to figuring out what it takes to get better.

But Mitzi is also quick to point out that what we're calling the All-Pro Diet can produce enormous benefits not just for athletes but for anyone. This is where her experience as a nutritionist comes in very handy. What if a 45-year-old woman, for instance, went on the All-Pro Diet? What difference would it make in *her* health? Or what about a guy who was the opposite of me in terms of lifestyle—instead of working out every day and going through intense practices and demanding games, what if he sat behind a desk for most of the day? Would the diet do any good?

Here's a quick analysis of the way Mitzi sized up the benefits.

As Mitzi notes, many women in their thirties, forties, and fifties struggle with weight gain, and because many are multitasking and have very demanding lifestyles, they often feel rundown and tired. On the All-Pro Diet, the change in eating patterns results, almost immediately, in weight loss and improved strength. A woman on this diet (and Mitzi is a good example!) will have increased steady energy levels, without the ragged highs and lows (in blood sugar as well as energy) that people get on a diet of high-fat, high-sugar, highly processed foods. There's greater enjoyment in eating foods closer to nature, and more energy derived from eating "clean" foods without artificial ingredients and added sodium. Anyone who goes on a diet like this one—with an emphasis on whole grains with moderate protein and plenty of fruits and vegetables with healthy fats—can avoid the stress to the pancreas resulting from diets high in sugar and refined carbohydrates. And many women, Mitzi says, will see an improvement in their skin. That's the result of eating more foods with omega-3s (these fatty acids are very good for the skin and help it look younger) and avoiding sugar and trans fats.

Men who go on the All-Pro Diet may begin with the goal of getting to a healthy weight while building muscle and losing fat. Those kinds of results come pretty quickly (especially if you follow the kind of workout routine I describe in Chapter 9). Since a lot of guys try to play down health concerns, they may be less aware of other powerful benefits of the All-Pro Diet, but as I pointed out earlier, all the studies point to clear rewards in terms of decreasing risks for obesity, diabetes, heart disease, stroke, cancer, and hypertension. And apart from all that, there's a lot to be said for really enjoying the food you're eating. When people in the habit of wolfing down a lot of food start being more selective—and just *slow down*—it's like getting their tastebuds back. We are what we eat, and when you eat more whole foods instead of relying on packaged foods high in artificial ingredients, you just feel better.

THE UPSIDE OF DAIRY CONTROL

When some people first look at the All-Pro Diet, they immediately notice how few dairy products are on the menu. As someone who loves milk, ice cream, and (especially) cheese, I thought it might be really difficult to give up these foods. At first, I went for a total ban, and with interesting results. I've always had sinus and breathing problems, but as soon as I eliminated

---

THE ALL-PRO DIET BENEFIT PACKAGE

In my view, the All-Pro Diet Benefit Package is the best health insurance package available today. And you can get it all at your local farmers' market, supermarket, health food store, and online. Plus, there's no additional cost. (In fact, you will likely *save* money in your food budget on this diet plan.) And as Mitzi points out, every one of these benefits is supported by leading research in health, diet, and nutrition.

On the All-Pro Diet, you will . . .

- Build muscle
- Lose fat
- Get lean
- Improve your energy levels
- Improve your complexion
- Improve your digestion
- Increase your eating enjoyment
- Greatly lower your risk of the diet-related killers—cancer, obesity, heart disease, diabetes, and hypertension

dairy, all of these problems cleared up. Again—coincidence? I don't think so, because as long as I've stayed off milk products or kept them to a minimum, my sinuses have stayed clear.

So, for me, that's an ongoing incentive to avoid dairy. But of course there are other reasons, not so tangible. Many dairy foods have high saturated fat content—that in itself is a problem. But in addition, we've become increasingly aware of how many children and adults have lactose intolerance, which means that dairy products can have a bad effect on the digestive system. (Cramping, gas, and diarrhea are common symptoms of lactose intolerance.) Research shows that approximately 75 percent of adults in the world do not make enough, or any, lactase—the enzyme responsible for breaking down lactose in dairy products.

One reason many people are reluctant to give up milk is the belief that it builds strong bones. While it's true that milk does have a great supply of calcium and therefore helps bone-building, there's something wrong with the concept that it's the only approach. The fact is, the United States has the

THE BOTTOM LINE ON DAIRY

"Despite what those splashy milk-mustache ads imply, dairy products are not a silver (or white) bullet to bone health. Can they be part of a healthy diet if you enjoy dairy and stick to low-fat and nonfat choices? Absolutely. But they certainly aren't a requirement for a healthy body. Consider that more than 75 percent of the world's population includes little or no dairy products at all in their diets. Secondly, when you look at the numbers, the countries with the lowest intakes of calcium in the world (for example, India and Japan have a daily intake of about 300 milligrams a day) have some of the lowest rates of hip fracture and osteoporosis, while people with some of the highest intakes (the United States and Finland have average intakes of at least 1,000 milligrams a day) also have the highest rates of osteoporosis."

—Kate Geagan, MS, RD, author of *Go Green, Get Lean:*
Trim Your Waistline with the Ultimate Low-Carbon Footprint Diet

highest rate of osteoporosis—the early bone loss that is particularly damaging to women—of any country in the world. And this is a country where advertising campaigns are constantly urging us to drink a lot of milk.

You can drink 1% low-fat organic milk on the All-Pro Diet if it agrees with your body. (And, by the way, Mitzi recommends organic chocolate milk as a recovery drink—especially for kids—because the protein to carbohydrate ratio is very good.) But I don't want you to think that the only way to have strong bones is by drinking three or four glasses of milk each day.

As for cheese, even though I love it, I definitely recommend that you cut back on high-fat cheeses. Their saturated fat, we know, contributes to heart

MITZI ADVISES: GET YOUR VITAMIN D

If you follow the news at all, you have likely seen a story about vitamin D. It's become the super vitamin. We know vitamin D plays an important role in the absorption of calcium for our bones and muscle strength, but recently there has been a lot more hype about other potential powers of vitamin D. Low blood levels of vitamin D have been linked to many diseases including: breast cancer, colon cancer, diabetes, and heart disease.

RECOMMENDATIONS

The Food and Nutrition Board currently recommends 200 international units (IU) of vitamin D for adults up to age 50. For adults older than 50, they recommend 400 to 600 IU. However, many vitamin D experts are now suggesting a daily intake of 800 to 1,000 IU. It is definitely a good idea to discuss vitamin D supplementation with your doctor.

FOOD SOURCES OF VITAMIN D

Vitamin D is naturally present in very few foods; however, some foods are fortified with vitamin D. Here is a list of vitamin D containing foods:

Cod liver oil	Fortified cereals (read the label)
Fortified milk	Some orange juice is also fortified with vitamin D
Salmon	

disease. Of course we all need calcium as well as other nutrients like vitamin D that contribute to bone-building. But as Mitzi points out, it's important to be aware that milk and other dairy products are *not* the only source of calcium. Keep in mind, adults under the age of 50 need 1,000 milligrams of calcium per day, while adults over the age of 50 need 1,200 milligrams of calcium per day. One cup of organic 1% milk provides about 300 milligrams of calcium. Some nondairy food sources of calcium include fortified cereals, salmon, sardines, fortified orange juice, and many dark, leafy green vegetables. I do take a calcium supplement to make sure I'm meeting my calcium goals.

YOU'LL NEED YOUR PROTEIN

As I mentioned earlier, I was on a completely vegan diet for a very short time, but I quickly realized I needed some additional protein sources. Personally, I prefer fish to chicken. But if you like chicken more, there's nothing wrong with broadening your diet that way. The goal is to have fish three to four times per week.

Red meat is not ideal. A recent study in the *Archives of Internal Medicine* suggests that people who eat more red meat and processed meat have a higher risk of death from cancer, heart disease, and other causes compared to those with lower intakes. The saturated fat found in red meat is also known to increase the risk of some types of cancer. But, according to Mitzi, a little beef is okay. On the All-Pro Diet, you should limit yourself to no more than 18 ounces per month. Also, when you do eat it, be selective. You want grass-fed beef: It's free of all the additives that appear when cows are given antibiotics and fed mountains of corn.

WHAT IS GRASS-FED AND GRASS-FINISHED MEAT?

One of the most interesting things I have learned on my nutrition journey has come from reading two books that Mitzi gave me, both by Michael Pollan—*In Defense of Food* and *The Omnivore's Dilemma*. I recommend you read them both. They definitely opened my eyes to how our current food system works and also helped me feel comfortable including a small amount of grass-finished meat in my diet on occasion.

Here's what I learned from Pollan and Mitzi: Most cows are grain-fed. They eat a concentrated feed made of corn and soybeans. This concentrated feed makes the cows grow fatter faster. Since cows were meant to eat grass, changing their diet in this way has some negative consequences. The USDA has yet to offer an official definition for grass-fed beef or grass-finished beef. Most grass-fed cows have eaten grass throughout their lives, but some grass-fed beef producers actually grain-feed their cattle during their last 90 to 160 days to fatten them up. This is why it is important to make sure the beef is actually "grass-finished": It means the cattle are finished on grass until the day of processing.

There are clear reasons for choosing grass-finished over grain-fed beef. Cows that are raised in feedlots have higher levels of harmful bacteria like E. coli and Campylobacter as well as dangerous bacteria in their feces. Grass-finished cows have a better omega-3 profile as well as other important nutrients found in grass, like vitamin E and conjugated linoleic acid, or CLA.

The bottom line is to aim for grass-finished meat. The majority of commercial beef as well as much organic or "natural" meat is finished with grain, often in confined feedlots. Your goal should be to buy meat with no hormones or antibiotics from humanely treated grass-fed and grass-finished animals.

SWITCHING OVER

Once you switch over from old eating habits and get on the All-Pro Diet, you want to stay there. That's why there's so much variety in the recipes, meals, and lists that Mitzi has created.

I love to eat! Food has been and always will be an enjoyable part of my life. In switching over from my old diet to the All-Pro Diet, I feel as though all changes have been positive ones—I get to eat food that I enjoy, I take more pleasure in the time I spend eating, and I've been able to savor a whole new range of flavors. Do I still have a small bowl of ice cream sometimes? Of course, but it's *rice* ice cream. Do I get a slice of my kid's birthday cake? Almost always, but minus the frosting! (Or, sometimes I choose an oatmeal raisin or a chocolate chip cookie instead of cake.) Those are foods that I also enjoy. But when I do that, I don't feel like someone's going to throw down the penalty flag. It's not like I'm "good" on the All-Pro Diet and "bad" when I have some other food that also happens to taste good. Sometimes I like to call an audible, change my game a little, and then go back to the All-Pro Diet again.

We want you to know that in this diet you can enjoy many of the foods you love. You don't need to have an all-or-nothing diet mentality. And why not? Because with that kind of mentality, you put too much pressure on yourself to eat "perfectly," and that's simply too difficult to maintain forever.

Here's the deal: I don't eat perfectly. Mitzi doesn't eat perfectly. The only difference is that we know how to balance it all. Our goal is to teach you that if you have a day of making unhealthy choices, you can, without hesitation, start over strong the next day. You just can't let too many days go by where you aren't paying attention to how you are fueling your body. We don't want to be the food police, but we do want to help guide you and your family toward a new way of eating. That's right. You should also be using the All-Pro Diet principles as the foundation for what to feed your kids to promote good health, optimal energy, and peak performance. I realize this may seem new to people who think of a diet as deprivation and feel like they're cheating when they go off it. But the mindset really is different. If you feel that you're cheating every time you have a little bowl of ice cream, then you start to associate cheating with holidays, vacation, or downtime.

A good example: Not long ago, I took a vacation with my brother, and he decided that as long as he was taking a break from work, he might as well take a break from a healthy diet. So, for 3 days, he was eating pasta in creamy sauces, burgers with cheese, and potatoes covered with dollops of sour cream. We hang out often enough that he knows about my interest in a mostly plant-based diet, and most of the time he tries to follow the same plan. But during this vacation, he was loading up on meat-focused meals laden with dairy products like butter, cheese, and sour cream and then telling me, "I don't normally eat like this!"

So—what's that supposed to mean? That vacations aren't "normal"? Well, maybe not, but on vacation you often have great opportunities to try out new foods that are still in line with the All-Pro Diet. My brother and I were in a place where he could have been trying out a wide variety of fresh fruits, vegetables, and grain dishes with unusual flavors, and instead he was choosing all kinds of foods that had caused him to be tired and have low energy levels in the past and were setting the stage for worsening health conditions in the future.

The point is, try to stick to the All-Pro Diet wherever you go, regardless of where you're traveling, what you're celebrating, or how you're vacationing. Keep looking out for new taste experiences, and by all means try interesting foods. That's the fun of eating—and pleasing your tastebuds! But while you're at it, go for foods that are in line with the 17 All-Pro Diet Principles that I outline in the next chapter. Once you get a knack for that, you'll be amazed at how many healthful foods are out there for you to enjoy.

> **"YOU MAY BE DISAPPOINTED IF YOU FAIL,**
> **BUT YOU ARE DOOMED IF YOU DON'T TRY."**
>
> —Beverly Sills, American Operatic Soprano

THE OLD AND THE NEW

On the All-Pro Diet, I'm a flexitarian. That means I'm primarily eating plant-based foods, but I still include fish, eggs, chicken, fish oils, and occasionally grass-finished meat. I do eat dairy on occasion (since cheese was the food I missed the most), and my recovery drink has whey protein, which is a milk-based product.

Here's a comparison between a typical day on my old diet and a typical day on my flexitarian All-Pro Diet. Mitzi has done a nutritional analysis for both days, so you can see the huge differences, particularly in my consumption of total fat, saturated fat, and cholesterol. And on the All-Pro Diet, I'm getting more than twice as much dietary fiber each day as I once was!

The Old Diet

BREAKFAST

Fried egg sandwich with bacon on 2 slices white bread

12 ounces whole milk

10 ounces orange juice

LUNCH

Hamburger with bacon

French fries

Milkshake

Water

DINNER

12-ounce rib eye steak

Mashed potatoes with butter and sour cream

Mixed vegetables in butter

Apple pie à la mode

Water

Total calories: 4,727

Protein: 211 g

Carbohydrates: 419 g

Total fat: 246 g

Saturated fat: 103 mg

Cholesterol: 1,134 mg

Fiber: 24 g

The All-Pro Diet

BREAKFAST

Tony's Morning Power Smoothie (recipe on page 124)

1½ cups steel-cut oatmeal with 2 tablespoons flaxseed and 1 tablespoon agave nectar

LUNCH

2 cups Black Bean Soup (recipe on page 137)

1 cup brown rice

1½ cups mixed vegetables

Water

SNACK

Raw Revolution energy bar

10.5-ounce bottle Sambazon Açaí Juice

DINNER

10 ounces grilled wild salmon

1 cup sautéed spinach

1½ cups whole wheat pasta with red sauce

1 cup raspberry sorbet

Water

Total calories: 3,497

Protein: 189 g

Carbohydrates: 511 g

Total fat: 86 g

Saturated fat: 7 mg

Cholesterol: 199 mg

Fiber: 53 g

GETTING WITH THE PROGRAM

Most people follow a diet for a short period of time, lose weight, go off the diet, and gain it all back. That's even more dangerous than being overweight. Constant weight fluctuation is tough on your entire body. The All-Pro Diet is not a 30-day experiment. I'm hoping that people can make it their day-to-day way of eating for health and success for the rest of their lives.

Mitzi points out that it usually takes people about 30 days to develop new eating habits. I think it can actually take a couple of months before the All-Pro Diet becomes totally second nature. It will take you some time to try out our recipes and find your favorites. That's why Mitzi has divided the introductory steps into two phases, so you won't have to do everything at once. Phase I of the program starts on page 101. As long as you make sure to get protein at each meal (as specified in the recipes), you will start to feel better within days. After about 2 weeks, you will really notice the difference. Once you move into Phase II (see page 108) and the habits you've developed in this program become automatic, there's no reason to ever turn back to your old diet.

MITZI'S TIPS FOR PERMANENT WEIGHT LOSS

I know my current diet will allow me to control my weight better as I get older and eventually retire from football. A lot of guys start gaining weight after they hit 30, but I tell people it is always possible to look and feel better than you did in your twenties. It will take some dedication and hard work, but nothing good in life comes easy. I've asked Mitzi to share some of her key weight-loss advice for helping both professional athletes as well as the average Joe.

If you are looking to lose weight, it's really a simple mathematical calculation. Your goal is to burn more calories than you consume—there are 3,500 calories in 1 pound of fat! By taking in 500 fewer calories each day, you should lose about 1 pound every 7 days.

There are three ways to lose weight: (1) Eat less. (2) Move more. (3) Do both! I typically suggest number 3, "Do both!" When an athlete is *already* doing extra work, that is, extra conditioning in addition to his or her strength program, then I know their difficulty to lose weight is 90 percent diet. For people who focus only on their workouts and follow them up with a big, juicy hamburger, french fries, and a soda, weight loss ain't gonna happen.

So, if you are working out but sabotaging your efforts with poor eating habits, you can make some simple changes to see your abs again. Each of these factors is essential if you're trying to get leaner and lose weight:

- Avoid drinking any juice, alcohol, or soda, and limit sports drinks to during and after exercise. (You can also make half portions of the recovery smoothies.)
- Decrease your portion sizes.
- Avoid cleaning your plate.
- Stop eating when you are satisfied; not full, stuffed, or sick.
- Don't eat while watching TV.
- Drink plenty of water.
- Avoid the all-or-nothing mentality.
- Eat a source of protein at every meal and combine with a small portion of whole grains.
- Avoid eating after 7:30 p.m.

By following the above steps in addition to our meal plans, you will definitely start losing weight. When you're on the All-Pro Diet, you will also notice that, in general, you retain less water, since you greatly reduce your intake of sodium-rich processed foods.

CHAPTER 3

THE 17 ALL-PRO DIET PRINCIPLES

"THE GREAT THING IN THIS WORLD IS NOT SO MUCH WHERE WE ARE, BUT IN WHAT DIRECTION WE ARE MOVING."

—Oliver Wendell Holmes Sr., American Physician and Author

The next step is focusing on the specific foods that you want in your personal plan. In the pages ahead, you'll find plenty of examples of delicious foods that you will enjoy for a lifetime as a part of your new whole foods eating plan. My goal is to help you create a personalized program that you can stick with to realize gains in health and wellness for the rest of your life. Then let's get down to the business of cleaning up your diet once and for all. Mitzi and I will show you the meal plans and recipes that will take you to the next level.

Not long ago, Mitzi and I started to make a list of what have become, for me, the essential principles of the All-Pro Diet. When we were done, there were just 17 items on that list. We realized then that many of these principles were quite simple. You might have to tweak your schedule at first and make some extra food-shopping trips, but if you gradually introduce these principles into your life, I think you'll find it to be a smooth transition.

So here they are.

MITZI AND TONY G'S TOP NUTRITION TIPS: OUR 17 ALL-PRO DIET PRINCIPLES

1. Eat lean protein and whole grains at every meal.

2. Eat every 3 to 4 hours.

3. Eat three meals and one to three snacks every day.

4. Eat plenty of fruits and vegetables every day.

5. Drink plenty of water.

6. Avoid foods with saturated and trans fats.

7. Avoid highly processed foods and foods with artificial ingredients.

8. Eat a diet high in omega-3s.

9. Avoid refined carbohydrates like white rice and white bread.

10. Practice portion control.

11. Stop eating as soon as you feel satisfied.

12. Avoid drinking your calories in the form of soda, juice, specialty coffee drinks, and alcoholic beverages.

13. Never skip a meal.

14. Avoid added sugars.

15. Avoid fast food.

16. Always eat a healthy breakfast.

17. Avoid eating after 7:30 p.m. when you're trying to lose weight.

Take a second look at this list. It might be worth asking yourself: If I could avoid a preventable death by following these guidelines, would I do it?

It's worth thinking about. After all, this is your health, and your health is your life.

Before we go any further, let's take a closer look at the 17 All-Pro Diet Principles—where they come from, why they're important, and how you can integrate them into your daily life and eating habits.

1. EAT LEAN PROTEIN AND WHOLE GRAINS AT EVERY MEAL.

Where does lean protein come from? There are a number of good sources. Protein is abundantly plentiful in fish, and, as I've noted, that's a regular part of my diet. Some fish is a little higher in fat, but that's actually a good thing. (We will talk more about omega-3s, also known as the "good fats," in a little bit.) I have fish about four times a week and chicken about two or three times a week. You can also get protein from nonanimal sources like quinoa, beans, lentils, fermented soy, and other kinds of supplements. (In our recommendations and recipes, we'll list a large number of sources.) There's also some protein in whole grains, which is just one reason they're an essential part of the All-Pro Diet.

As I've mentioned, I did try a strictly vegan regimen for a while. Frankly, I went off that diet because it wasn't enabling me to get the most out of my body on the football field. As I lost weight and strength, Mitzi advised me that I needed to increase my protein intake. I was wary at first, because Dr. Campbell had identified what he believed to be many of the shortcomings of protein in the diet. What turned me around was the clear fact that I wouldn't be able to cut it as an elite athlete if I continued to lose weight and strength. I needed protein if I was going to perform at my absolute best.

The turnaround came one weekend when I met Jon Hinds, a mostly vegan trainer Dr. Campbell introduced to me. He owns Monkey Bar Gym in Madison, Wisconsin. Jon and his wife came to the Kansas City Chiefs' training camp in Wisconsin, and they taught me how to shop for healthy foods like whole grain breads. He also taught me how to make protein shakes with spinach, cherries, and açaí (a wild berry grown in the Amazon rain forest). Jon showed me how to combine pea protein, rice protein, and hemp protein for a tremendous energy boost. Almost immediately, I felt a huge improvement. (Be sure to check out my delicious protein shake recipe—Tony's Morning Power Smoothie—on page 124.)

2. EAT EVERY 3 TO 4 HOURS.

Did you just do a double take? Wasn't it just a few pages ago that I was warning about all the dangerous consequences of obesity? And now Mitzi and I are advising you to eat every 3 to 4 hours?

Ah, yes. But of course I'm *not* talking about grabbing fast food or packaged snacks when you're on the go. To get the benefit of this particular principle in the All-Pro Diet, you have to integrate it with our other recommendations (particularly principles 11 through 14). Understandably, your energy levels are bound to go up and down during the day. By eating more frequently—every 3 to 4 hours throughout the day—you're giving your body a more steady supply of nutrients. Also, your hunger doesn't build up to the point where you feel really famished and are ready to eat almost anything.

If you follow principle 2, I can guarantee you will never feel hungry as long as you eat the right combinations of food, which include sources of protein, whole grains, and fruits and vegetables.

3. EAT THREE MEALS AND ONE TO THREE SNACKS EVERY DAY.

On pages 77–122, you'll find great recommendations for many of the meals that Mitzi has created for the All-Pro Diet. I've already shown you what one day of meals looks like for me, but of course I'm taking in a lot more calories than you need. Just to give you a quick preview, here's what your day of meals and snacks might look like:

For breakfast, you might start off with one packet of Nature's Path Hot Oatmeal or 1 cup cooked steel-cut oatmeal made with water, ½ cup of blueberries, and 1 scoop protein powder. (I like to have a cup of green tea to go along with that.) Later in the morning, for a snack, have a handful (about ½ cup) of raw almonds and dried cranberries along with a very small piece (1 ounce) of salmon jerky. For lunch, follow Mitzi's delicious recipe for Black Beans with Quinoa (page 151): It's delicious served with 10 baby carrots. Afternoon snack is a Raw Revolution energy bar along with green tea. For dinner, I might choose Fish Tacos (page 149), Easy Asparagus (page 155), and 1 ounce of dark chocolate. And the day's total is 1,809 calories, 109 grams of protein, 228 grams of carbohydrates, and 57 grams of fat.

Of course, every day's menu is different—and the more variety, the better. But you can see from this example how it's possible to have three terrific meals and a number of tasty snacks during the day without going overboard. And you won't get hungry. If you take your time eating, by eating more slowly and more consciously, I think you'll find that you feel pleasantly well-fed—without feeling overstuffed—throughout the day.

4. EAT PLENTY OF FRUITS AND VEGETABLES EVERY DAY.

In the day of meals I described above, you'll notice there were servings of blueberries, cranberries, carrots, and asparagus in addition to grains, legumes, nuts, whole grains, fish, pasta, and beverages. Of all those dietary elements, fruits and vegetables rank extremely high in nutrients. If I were to give you a list of all the nutrients contained in fruits and vegetables alone—including the fiber that contributes so much to digestive health—the list would fill an entire page. But as nutritionists have come to understand, even the full list of nutritional components does not begin to tell the whole story. Fruits are loaded with disease-fighting antioxidants and phytochemicals. It may be many years before scientists completely understand the benefits that come from eating lots of fruit and vegetables—and in the meantime, all we know is what happens when people live on a diet that deprives them of the unique combination of naturally occurring ingredients that are clearly essential to life and health. As a general rule of thumb, aim to eat about 2 cups of fruit and 2½ cups of vegetables per day.

5. DRINK PLENTY OF WATER.

The formula: Calculate your daily fluid requirement by dividing your bodyweight by 2. That number is the number of ounces of water you need to consume each and every day to stay hydrated.

To athletes, the habit of staying hydrated is almost second nature. Coming off the field, we reach for that water bottle. Tennis players rehydrate between sets. Long-distance runners get their doses before, during, and after the run. Athletes know how rapidly water evaporates from their bodies in the heat of activity, and our parched throats remind us that it's time to gulp another few ounces.

But what are the reminders when you're indoors most of the day, working in an office, sitting in front of a computer, or operating machinery? At low levels of activity, you don't get that parched feeling. After a couple of cups of coffee or tea in the morning and some kind of beverage at noon, you may feel as if your body has all the fluid it needs.

Dehydration can sneak up on you, significantly lowering your energy levels and, in fact, impeding a lot of normal body processes. The body, after all, is made up largely of water, and water is what it needs for nerves and muscles as well as the heart, kidneys, liver, bladder, and the entire digestive system to function well.

The formula above is the simplest I've seen—and it works. If your body weight is 160 pounds, you'll need 80 ounces of water each day to stay hydrated. That's 5 pints or 10 cups. For me, at 246 pounds, it's closer to 8 pints or 16 cups a day minimum. No matter where I am, I almost always have a bottle of water within reach.

Of course, you're also getting hydrated with other beverages. Coffee, tea, milk, and sports drinks count as fluids. It is true that the caffeine in coffee can act as a mild diuretic, but it is not enough to discount it as a fluid. In the end, water is the easiest, cheapest, and most direct source of the fluids you need. Your body depends on it.

6. AVOID FOODS WITH SATURATED AND TRANS FATS.

These two kinds of fat are the big-time culprits in many cases of heart attack and stroke. With very few exceptions, people who consistently load up on fatty meat and meat products (like hot dogs, sausage, and hamburgers) are at a higher risk of heart disease than people who trade off with fruits, vegetables, grains, and legumes that have little or no saturated fat. Whole milk and cheese are very high in saturated fat. So, right there, you can see why we significantly reduce those foods in the All-Pro Diet.

There's been so much bad press about foods with saturated fat that most people realize by now the serious health risks in a diet that features lots of fatty meat, butter, eggs, and ice cream. What has been harder to get across is the risk of trans fats. These have long been used by food packagers to help preserve products. Trans fats are created when food manufacturers add hydrogen to vegetable oil (a process called hydrogenation) in order to increase shelf life and prevent spoilage. For many years, it was thought that trans fats were relatively harmless. They were created in the processing of thousands of brands of packaged foods, from crackers and cookies to vegetable shortening and margarine. Trans fats were also in the deep-fry cookers used to make french fries, particularly in fast-food restaurants.

It's now known that trans fat is a major contributor (along with saturated fat) to coronary heart disease. In fact, in a review of the research that he summarizes in his latest book, *In Defense of Food,* Michael Pollan concludes, "Trans fat is really bad stuff, apparently, fully twice as bad as saturated fat in its impact on cholesterol ratios." By contributing to the rise in LDL levels—low-density lipoprotein, the "bad" cholesterol in the bloodstream—it's reasonable to assume that trans fat is now implicated in the coronary heart disease deaths of millions of people.

The punishment for food manufacturers? There is none. But at least the Food and Drug Administration requires that trans fat be listed on the labels of packaged foods. "With the addition of trans fat to the nutrition fact panel," advises the FDA in its official announcement, "you can review your food choices and see how they stack up."

In plainer English, there's nothing to review. If you see trans fat listed on the food label, return the package to its place on the store shelf. A food label may show 0 gram trans fat per serving, but it may contain up to 0.49 gram of trans fat per serving. Avoid foods with "partially hydrogenated vegetable oil" and anything that includes the word "hydrogenated." Its contents do not belong in your body.

7. AVOID HIGHLY PROCESSED FOODS AND FOODS WITH ARTIFICIAL INGREDIENTS.

As I've said, food scientists don't really understand the special combination of nutritional properties in fruits and vegetables that make them such naturally good bodybuilders. Still less do they understand what exactly happens to food through the various processes of preserving and packaging that creates the edible content on your supermarket shelves. Nearly all the artificial ingredients added as coloring, flavoring, and preservatives are tested in laboratories, and it's a pretty sure bet that they won't poison you. In fact, many of the most common preservatives have undergone very close scrutiny by food scientists in the government and in the corporations that rely on food-processing and manufacturing for their business. The trouble is, *not poisonous* is quite different from *not harmful*. And, as I've just noted in the case of trans fats, scientists often do not understand the long-term effects of the added chemicals and elaborate processes used to maintain freshness and flavor.

Apart from the possibility of the long-term health risks of eating a lot of processed foods, there is also—and this is just as important—the loss-of-opportunity factor. Every time you eat a chip, cracker, or biscuit that was created from a stew of artificial and natural ingredients, stamped out by a machine, baked en masse, and poured into a bag, box, or wrapper, you are missing the opportunity to eat a grape, an almond, a slice of orange, a carrot, or a piece of apple. Think about it: Why would anyone want to do this? That fresh food in your left hand has an incredible combination of nutrients that took millennia to develop through a process of natural selection in the plant world, and it's a food that has been proven over generations to provide the sustenance for human life. The manufactured chip, cracker, or cookie in your right hand was made in a food laboratory, where scientists mixed the most recently developed preservative compounds with whatever ingredients were available to create a taste and texture that would survive many weeks in a package on a shelf and would invite you (the consumer) to eat so much that you never wanted to stop.

Left hand or right hand? Which do you choose?

Sounds like a no-brainer. But not so fast. If you *really* want to make that choice, there are several things you have to do, and these first steps may be tougher than they sound.

A POSITIVE GENETIC CHANGE

Making wise lifestyle choices can have an effect on your genes, according to a study published in the journal *Proceedings of the National Academy of Sciences.* Dr. Dean Ornish at the University of California, San Francisco, led a small study that showed a diet high in fruits, vegetables, legumes, and whole grains; exercise (for example, walking for 30 minutes a day); and an hour of stress management each day (for example, meditating) actually changed about 500 genes in the 30 male subjects. Some genes were turned off while others were turned on. While further studies will certainly be done, it looks like when you improve your lifestyle, you can improve your genes.

First, you have to find the *unpackaged* food in the supermarket—and that means hunting around the perimeter of the store where you'll find fruits and vegetables—the less-traveled areas where bargains and specials are not heavily advertised.

Second, when you see or hear a mouthwatering commercial for an incredibly tasty food—and you witness happy, beautiful people in those commercials having the time of their lives—you have to say to yourself, with all the cynicism of a Gen-Xer, "That's all hype!"

And, third, you have to give your tastebuds a chance. If you love eating chips, cookies, or crackers for that instant rush of highly manufactured flavor they provide, you'll need to approach the fresh food in your left hand with some understanding and patience. When you bite into an almond, enjoy the crunch, the subtle flavor. Take time to chew the whole thing before you swallow, to release the oils and phytonutrients that got their flavor from the soil and sun during months of cultivation. You can pop an orange slice into your mouth, chew it twice, and it'll be gone—*or* you can squeeze out the juice between your teeth, relish the pure orange flavor (unadvertised—but it's there!), and slowly chew the membrane that delivers healing fiber to your entire intestinal system.

Call that hard work? I don't. These days, I call it eating. Real food. It's delicious stuff.

8. EAT A DIET HIGH IN OMEGA-3S.

Ever since I started paying more attention to my diet, I've gotten an important but very rudimentary education in a rather obscure subject—fats. Rudimentary, because I still can't sling around the terms that doctors and food scientists love to use, and I'm not clear about the difference between a single and a double bond in a carbon chain. But I do know, at this point, some of the distinctions among bad, good, better, and best fats. And in this pecking order, omega-3 fatty acids are just about as good as fat gets.

Omega-3 fats (and omega-6 fats) are polyunsaturated fats (PUFAs) and cannot be made by your body: They must be consumed in your diet. While trans fats and most saturated fats are harmful due to their link to heart disease and obesity, omega-3s and omega-6s are essential to your health. According to Mitzi, most Americans get too much omega-6 and not enough omega-3. Our goal ratio should be somewhere between 1:1 (that is, the same amount of omega-6 as omega-3) and 3:1 (three times as much omega-6 as omega-3). Contrast that ideal ratio with what we usually get in our unbalanced Western diet, a ratio of about 20:1. That's way too much omega-6! That's because the vegetable-oil industry is flourishing, and much of that oil comes from seeds that are high in omega-6 fats. With the ratio so off kilter, we need to include more omega-3s to create a better balance. Omega-3s, however, are not so easy to come by, which is why Mitzi consistently recommends foods high in omega-3 content.

What are the benefits of omega-3s? Research shows that omega-3 fats are especially important in preventing heart disease. They do this by inhibiting the formation of blood clots, which can get stuck in blood vessels leading to the heart; decreasing your risk of deadly heartbeat abnormalities; and inhibiting or slowing the growth of plaques that narrow arteries.

In addition, research has revealed a growing list of diseases and conditions that are affected positively by omega-3s. That list includes the following:

- Decreasing hypertension (high blood pressure)
- Lowering triglyceride (harmful fat) levels in the blood
- Decreasing joint tenderness and inflammation around joints, which can be helpful for many people, including professional athletes, active people, and those suffering from rheumatoid arthritis
- Decreasing age-related memory loss and cognitive function impair-

ment; showing benefits for those with attention deficit disorder and bipolar disorder; and possibly lowering the risk for Alzheimer's disease

- Playing a role in preventing depression (A low level of omega-3s has been linked to depression.)

If I were in a huddle, with a goal of lifetime good health, and the quarterback said, "Omega-3s," I'd say it was a good call.

As I've noted, in the All-Pro Diet, Mitzi has put together a plan that will help you achieve the optimum ratio of omega-3 and omega-6 fats. Omega-3 fats consist of eicosapentaenoic acid (EPA), docosahexaenoic acid (DHA), and alpha-linolenic acid (ALA). Plant-based foods contribute omega-3s (ALA) through flaxseeds, flaxseed oil, and walnuts (although ALA is only partially converted to the important EPA and DHA). Typically, fish and often fish oil supplements are necessary if you're going to get enough omega-3s.

The best food sources? Topping the list is a number of different kinds of fish. The following table shows some other food sources as well.

Omega-3 Fatty Acid Content of Foods

Food Item	EPA grams	DHA grams	ALA grams
Salmon (3.5 oz)	0.8	0.6	
Tuna (3.5 oz)	0.3	0.9	
Swordfish (3.5 oz)	0.1	0.5	
Flaxseed oil (1 Tbsp)			7.5
Flaxseeds, ground (2 Tbsp)			3.5
Walnuts (1 oz, about 14 halves)			7.5
Soybeans, boiled (1½ cups)			0.5

This table explains why Mitzi recommends that I have fish about three to four times a week. I'm happy to do that—not only because I love fish but because it's such a great source of protein (see principle 1 again) and it delivers the benefits of a terrific omega-3 package.

However, be mindful of how often you are eating fish, since scientists are finding elevated mercury levels in some fish and fish products. It's highest in fish that consume other fish (leading to a buildup of mercury in their bodies). These include varieties like shark, swordfish, king mackerel, and tilefish—none of which are the most popular fish on the menu. If you are eating fish most days of the week, I would definitely suggest you get your mercury levels tested.

More typical on the American menu are canned fish like albacore (white) tuna and skipjack (light) tuna. Due to its smaller size, light tuna contains one-third the amount of mercury as albacore tuna. Environmental Protection Agency guidelines for women who are pregnant or plan to become pregnant state that it's safe to eat up to 12 ounces of light tuna a week or 6 ounces of white tuna a week (the standard weight of a can of tuna is 6 ounces). There is currently no recommended serving size for the general population. You can actually visit the Environmental Working Group's Web site at www.ewg.org/tunacalculator to calculate how much tuna is safe for you to eat. Researchers say you may be putting yourself at risk for mercury poisoning if you eat too much tuna and other fish containing mercury. Therefore, Mitzi suggests switching from fish with

MITZI ADVISES . . .

The risk of mercury-related problems is highest among pregnant women and very young women who eat a diet that includes lots of fish that has been contaminated. During pregnancy, very high levels of mercury can affect the fetus and have been linked to mental retardation and other health issues. Mercury poisoning in adults can cause numbness in fingers and toes, memory and vision loss, and tremors. It's very unlikely you'll find yourself experiencing any of these symptoms, but if you do, you need to visit your health care provider as soon as possible.

high mercury levels to other types of fish or seafood that don't contain as much mercury, such as salmon, sole, shrimp, herring, or haddock. Avoid eating shark and swordfish. Visit the following FDA Web site to find mercury levels of different species of fish: www.cfsan.fda.gov/~frf/ sea-mehg.html.

Since omega-3s provide so many benefits for heart health, the American Heart Association (AHA) has come out with a number of fish recommendations. If you're not meeting these requirements from food sources, Mitzi suggests taking fish-oil supplements to optimize your intake of fish oils (as well as minimize mercury intake). However, if you take 3 to 4 grams of fish oil in a day, this level can have potential blood-thinning effects, so always discuss any fish oil supplementation with your physician.

The AHA outlines the following:

- Healthy adults should consume fatty fish twice a week.
- Individuals with coronary heart disease should consume 1,000 milligrams of EPA plus DHA daily from oily fish. (Consult your physician about taking supplements to meet these levels.)
- Individuals with hypertriglyceridemia who are under a physician's care might benefit from taking 2 to 4 grams of EPA plus DHA per day—but they should consult with a doctor first.

Of course, as mentioned, there are dietary sources of omega-3s other than fish, though none are quite as stellar. Flaxseeds, flaxseed oil, and walnuts are high in alpha-linolenic acid (ALA), which is one of the three musketeers among the oils that make up omega-3s. Eggs from free-range chickens have higher amounts of omega-3s, and so does grass-finished beef. But these are also sources of saturated fats (in the "bad fat" category), so I'd never rely on eggs or beef as a significant omega-3 food source. Today, many foods have added omega-3s. And that's definitely a good thing. Every little bit helps!

9. AVOID REFINED CARBOHYDRATES LIKE WHITE RICE AND WHITE BREAD.

What's the matter with white rice and white bread?

If you'd grown up in the previous century, you would have regarded these foodstuffs as great luxuries and considered them a whole cut above plain brown rice or whole wheat bread. But there's a problem that we didn't anticipate back then. Refined white flour is essentially shorn of all the nutritious ingredients that are in the whole grain, and this is what goes into white bread (as well as into most cakes, cookies, and crackers). The same happens when brown rice is made into white rice. Nearly all the nutrients disappear during processing, and you're left with a food that your body very quickly turns to glucose (blood sugar). And that means your pancreas has to work overtime trying to *control* your blood sugar. Not only that, but whenever you fill up on these foods, you're missing a lot of the nutrients that the human body thrives on—like B vitamins, protein, and fiber. So if you're filling up on these kinds of foods, you're getting a lot of glucose but not much else. And your body needs a lot of other nutrients if it's going to thrive on the food you eat.

Among the white-flour products to avoid Mitzi also includes pasta, breads, bagels, wraps, pancakes, and pitas. Just look for whole grain versions instead. (Of course, there are times when you may be eating out at a restaurant that doesn't have whole grains. That's okay on occasion, but we don't want to see any of these in your pantry.) In general, your carbohydrates should come primarily from fruits, vegetables, and whole grains instead of sugar-laden foods and refined carbs. You want your carbs to be nutrient-rich foods instead of empty calories.

10. PRACTICE PORTION CONTROL.

For years, fast-food and chain restaurants have been trying to lure customers through their doors with offers of ever-increasing portion sizes. And it works! When people see mounds of food, you often hear things like "What a bargain!" followed by "I don't know if I can eat all that." But just as often, you'll hear people at the end of the meal saying, "I can't believe I finished all that." And right then, the waitperson appears to say, "How about dessert, everybody?"

Sound familiar? The fact is, many of us, whether we eat out a lot or a little, subscribe to the "clean plate club." We don't feel like we're finished until our plates are clean.

Well, if that's your operating mode, the only clear solution is portion control. If you look at the recipes that Mitzi includes in this book, you'll notice that she's very specific about portion sizes. When you start to follow this plan, it may seem at first as if you're depriving yourself. Not so! If anyone were to feel deprived, I'd be a pretty good candidate—and it just doesn't happen. I do clean my plate—as conscientiously as any little kid. But there's *less* on the plate I'm cleaning. And because I'm eating foods that are high in nutrients, and they're providing all the fuel I need to play the game at my best, I never feel like I'm getting shortchanged. The other good news is when you switch to a primarily whole foods diet, you eat a lot of fruits and vegetables that add volume without adding as many calories.

I *do* stay away from those fast-food restaurants, though. The food they mound on those plates is no bargain. Every time you clean a plate that's filled with that kind of food, there's a high price to pay in terms of health.

And that's the reason for the next principle on the list.

11. STOP EATING AS SOON AS YOU FEEL SATISFIED.

The trick here is patience. When we eat quickly, we often have no idea how full we are. That's because it takes time for the nerve endings around your stomach to start sending out signals that your mind interprets as "I'm full!" and "I've had enough."

Interestingly, researchers have actually discovered *how long* it takes for those all-done signals to reach the brain. That means if you stop to have a quick daily special at the nearest restaurant, there's a good chance you won't have any idea whether you're full or not when the waitperson comes back to ask whether you want dessert. The only way to know would be to wait at least 20 minutes, when you'll have some information based on real input from those nerve endings in your midsection. Needless to say, most of us are in too big a hurry for that.

So—what if you make it your assignment to stop eating when you feel satisfied? Well, first you'll become more aware of whether or not you're satisfied. Next, you'll eat more slowly, allowing more time for those all-important "all-done" signals to get to your brain, telling you when it's time to stop.

12. AVOID DRINKING YOUR CALORIES IN THE FORM OF SODA, JUICE, SPECIALTY COFFEE DRINKS, AND ALCOHOLIC BEVERAGES.

As Mitzi emphasizes, it's important to get plenty of fluids—but that's not where your calories should come from. High-calorie drinks certainly get glucose into your system, but you'll encounter the same problem as when eating a lot of any other kind of refined carbohydrate. Those drinks contain, for the most part, nutrient-free calories, which means your pancreas is challenged to process all that extra blood sugar, and the fat cells in your body are overfed (that is, you get fatter).

Most of us know about the consequences of drinking a lot of high-calorie soda. You're basically giving yourself a multi-teaspoon dose of sugar. One 20-ounce bottle of soda, for instance, is loaded with the equivalent of roughly 17 teaspoons of sugar in the form of high-fructose corn syrup. So . . . should you switch to diet soda, which has zero calories? It's not quite so simple because of the potential side effects of the sweeteners used in most of these sodas. In a recent study, the Atherosclerosis Risk in Communities, conducted by Dr. Lyn M. Steffen and her colleagues at the University of Minnesota's School of Public Health, researchers found a strong correlation between drinking diet soda and the metabolic syndrome I mentioned earlier that signals risk of cardiovascular disease and diabetes. The study showed a surprising 34 percent higher risk of developing metabolic syndrome among people who drank one can of diet soda a day compared with those who drank none.

Consuming fruit drinks also increases the risk of diabetes. A study published in the *Archives of Internal Medicine* showed women who drank two or more fruit drinks a day increased their risk by 31 percent compared to those who consumed less than one fruit drink a month. And other studies have shown a link between the consumption of fruit juice and diabetes. You're just much better off getting the same calories from whole fruits and vegetables.

As for coffee, if you drink it black, it's so low in calories that it's considered noncaloric. The trouble is, many people add more than a little cream and sugar. And when you consume one of the Starbucks-style specialty drinks, the calorie content becomes astronomical. A *venti* Iced White Chocolate Mocha with whipped cream, for instance, will set you back a whopping 630 calories, with 27 grams of fat, 18 grams of which are saturated.

With alcohol, there are really two problems. First, the calories are empty—they have almost no nutritional value at all. And second, it has a notoriously bad effect on the liver. That's because after you take a drink of alcohol, your body absorbs it into your bloodstream and it travels to the liver to be broken down. While your liver is busy metabolizing the alcohol, its ability to metabolize fat is suppressed. That delays the fat-burning process, leading to greater fat storage. And to make matters even worse, if you are consuming high carbohydrate alcoholic drinks, your body won't be able to burn the carbs until the alcohol is metabolized. The bottom line is to stay away from alcohol as much as possible when you are trying to lose body fat. (Alcohol contains 7 calories per gram; almost double that of both protein and carbohydrates at 4 calories per gram.)

Of course, the other notorious problem with alcohol is that it can be difficult to drink in moderation. After you knock back a few beers, you don't care as much about your diet and getting leaner. Then you kill a few more, and before you know it, you're eating (as well as drinking) a lot more than you ever meant to.

13. NEVER SKIP A MEAL.
I know guys who pride themselves on being able to keep working right through lunch or dinnertime, claiming, "It doesn't matter—I'm not hungry anyway." Well, maybe not. But just as you can be oblivious to the fact that you're full, you can be just as blind to the nutritional needs of your body throughout the day.

Missing a meal may seem like a minor oversight—or convenience—but there's sure to be an impact on your metabolism. When you don't have lunch, what happens to your energy level in mid or late afternoon? Your body is lacking its fuel supply, but more often than not, we say to ourselves, "I just need a quick cup of coffee to get me going again," or "Since I didn't have lunch, I guess it won't matter if I have a candy bar or two." Yes, you may feel a sudden surge after an energizing drink or snack, but you've initiated a whole new pattern of ups and downs in your energy, blood sugar levels, and metabolism. Instead of drawing on a steady sup-

MITZI ADVISES . . .

According to a study in the journal *Obesity*, people consistently eat more on the weekends. The best approach to weekend eating is planning ahead. If you are out and about all day, then pack some food to take with you. If you spend a lot of time at home, keep yourself busy with activities other than visiting your kitchen and eating all day.

ply of nutrients to provide an even distribution of energy throughout your day, your energy pattern turns into a ragged series of those ups and downs—deprivation followed by a surge of hunger—and you're sure to end up overeating in order to compensate.

14. AVOID ADDED SUGARS.

A lot of the guys on my team will eat two or three cookies at the end of lunch, which comes right after practice. We're not talking about little sugar wafers, either. These cookies are huge! I'm guessing 4 inches in diameter. The guys go crazy over them.

One day last season the cookies weren't set out at the beginning of lunch. Instead, they came out a little late, and it looked like a herd of cattle was going for the cookie basket. You would have thought the guys were homeless and hadn't eaten a meal in days.

It was good for a laugh, but when you look at the bigger picture, this hunger for added sugar starts to look pretty serious. The average American consumes about 31 teaspoons of *added* sugar every day. That means 117 pounds of added sugar per year!

One teaspoon of sugar has about 16 calories. When you multiply that by the average amount of added sugar consumed in a day, that's 500 sugar calories! Compare that with the recommendations from the World Health Organization, which say that your sugar intake should be 10 percent or less of total calories. For a person on a 2,220-calorie diet, that would mean getting no more than 55 grams of sugar in a day!

On the All-Pro Diet, the recommendation is even less. We want to shift your diet away from added sugars like refined white sugar and high-fructose corn syrup, which can actually increase your cravings for sweets. Does this mean you can no longer enjoy your favorite dessert? Not at all! Just this: You really don't need a 4-inch chocolate chip cookie every day . . . or two or three of them every day!

15. AVOID FAST FOOD.

If the way I portrayed myself at the beginning of this book makes me sound like I was a fast-food fanatic, that's pretty close to the truth. To me it was nothing to go in and order a couple of Whoppers with cheese, a large order of fries, and a supersized shake. I ate fast, hardly tasting my food, and I was so into sports, I thought I could always work it off, no problem.

I think that's the attitude most of us have when we get that sudden urge to grab a meal. It'll be ready in minutes, we'll eat fast, and we're so busy, we can't help but burn up those calories pretty quickly.

The only trouble is, we don't think much about how that food is prepared, what has to be done to it before it even enters the microwave or deep fryer. There's a huge difference between a meal packaged by manufacturers and sold by the millions and a single serving that you prepare from whole, fresh foods in your kitchen. Without sitting down to work out a careful nutritional analysis, it all comes down to this: Fast-food meals are mass-produced. And when food is mass-produced, it emerges stripped of some of the qualities that made it food in the first place. So as you eat more mass-produced food, you get comparatively fewer nutrients and more artificial ingredients. Your body gets what it doesn't need— usually all kinds of trans and saturated fats—in exchange for what it does need, which is quality fuel.

16. ALWAYS EAT A HEALTHY BREAKFAST.

When I realized that a healthy breakfast did not mean the same thing as a hearty breakfast, I started to reevaluate those bacon-and-egg extravaganzas that used to start my day. But as I discussed with Mitzi what would make a good breakfast, I realized that I really liked to have variety in this meal. She created a number of delicious smoothies that you'll find in the recipes in Chapter 7. In addition, I sometimes like to start my day with a bowl of oatmeal or granola with macadamia nuts. (However, instead of adding brown sugar or refined sugar, I'll use agave nectar—a great natural sweetener.) Another breakfast option is nondairy waffles with real organic maple syrup. (I'll never buy any syrup that has high-fructose corn syrup.) And I like whole wheat toast with Earth Balance Natural Buttery Spread—a nondairy butter.

17. AVOID EATING AFTER 7:30 P.M. WHEN YOU'RE TRYING TO LOSE WEIGHT.

If you're an active person and I've sold you on the other principles in this list, there's a very good chance that any weight-gain challenges you've had in the past will be completely under control. You'll be on a steady diet without the ragged ups and downs that are created by large doses of refined carbohydrates, and you'll find that your appetite is satisfied by the variety and range of foods in this plan. But there is one more key to weight loss—and for many, I'm afraid, it means breaking out of a pattern.

If an after-dinner or late-night snack has become a habit, it could be a tough one to break. The trouble is, this is the time of day when you're winding down, and there could be a whole lot of reasons, completely unrelated to appetite, why you want a little something before you go to bed. When we're tired, bored, stressed, or depressed, we sometimes look for something to eat when, really, the only thing to do is put our head on a pillow and relax.

Also, the postdinner hours are often spent watching TV, an activity during which munching chips or cookies can easily become an unconscious habit. But with bedtime not far away, it means we're not about to do anything in the next dozen or so hours that will burn the calories. So what we eat, late in the evening, is usually excessive. And that excess soon begins to build up in very visible ways—on stomach, hips, and thighs. As Mitzi explains, eating right before bed is an easy way to sabotage weight loss efforts, because instead of burning fat, your body is busy trying to metabolize all the calories you just fed it.

FOLLOWING THE PRINCIPLES

The great thing about the All-Pro Diet is that when you start to follow these 17 principles and begin making the recipes Mitzi has created, you'll feel the difference almost instantly. As soon as I changed my breakfast routine and started drinking the terrific shakes with high-nutrition ingredients that Mitzi recommends, I noticed that my strength improved. With the addition of fish and chicken to my diet, along with other concentrated sources of the protein I needed, I was back to lifting heavy weights and enjoying productive workouts. Beans and lentils turned out to be another protein boost, and I noticed that they pumped me up with even more strength and energy.

Now that I've completely switched over to the All-Pro Diet, I look forward to every meal and snack of the day. Once you're in the swing of things, the diet really doesn't take a whole lot of planning. It's just a matter of having the appropriate high-nutrition foods on hand, figuring out where you can get the best food when you eat out, understanding that it is not an all-or-nothing approach, and keeping to the 17 All-Pro Diet Principles.

CHAPTER 4

PREPARE FOR THE HIKE

"IF YOU WANT TO GET SOMEWHERE YOU HAVE TO KNOW WHERE YOU WANT TO GO AND HOW TO GET THERE. THEN NEVER, NEVER, NEVER GIVE UP."

—Norman Vincent Peale, author of *The Power of Positive Thinking*

In the All-Pro Diet, there are a few key nutrition basics that you'll need to appreciate before you begin. I'm going to summarize them in this chapter to help you calculate some of your personal dietary requirements and preferences. I'll also list some of the basic kitchen tools and ingredients you'll need to get started on the All-Pro Diet.

I want to emphasize one thing before we start, though. As I've said, this diet is not just for athletes or just for me. It really is for everyone. Whether you're the active type or you sit at a desk all day, this plan will work. Entire families should be eating this way. You just can't beat the benefits.

With this diet, you'll notice that Mitzi and I are not trying to turn you into a superstrict calorie counter. In fact, even though we've included calorie information as a reference point, you'll be okay as long as you're eating the right foods most of the time and watching your portions. This diet is more about paying attention to your hunger and satiety cues. When you've eaten enough to be satisfied, *that's* when you stop eating! It is possible to eat too much even if you are picking the right foods. With the All-Pro Diet, you can work toward a weight-loss goal as well as a health goal without careful calorie-counting, and on top of that, you can really enjoy what you're eating. Research does show that most people who have successfully lost weight and maintained the weight loss keep a food record. For a free downloadable All-Pro Diet food log, visit www.theallprodiet.com.

But, again, don't plan on doing this all at once. Like I said before, *you have to slow down before you turn around!*

BACK TO YOUR PROTEIN FUTURE

As soon as Mitzi and I began working on the All-Pro Diet, we realized that, in large part, the success of the program would depend on getting enough protein. Protein is crucial to maintaining optimal energy, and I work so hard during my workouts and on the field, I can't afford to get shortchanged, even for a single day. If you embrace this program as I hope you will, it's essential to figure out, right at the outset, how much protein you'll require in your new and improved daily nutritional regimen. (If you have compromised kidney function or you are on a protein-restricted diet, be sure to talk with your physician before you begin following the protein recommendations in the All-Pro Diet; it might have to be modified to fit your health profile.)

Many people refer to the federal guidelines for Recommended Dietary Allowances (RDA) suggesting that the daily intake of protein should be 0.36 gram per pound for individuals over the age of 18. That's the current RDA recommendation. According to Mitzi, though, research has shown that this isn't enough for active individuals. Physically active people and professional athletes have higher protein needs, and it's essential to meet those needs in order to build and repair muscle.

Protein is a very important food nutrient, as it helps build muscle and burn fat. (It helps increase the thermic effect of food, meaning that it helps boost metabolism.) Elevating protein intake also helps preserve lean muscle mass while decreasing body fat and promotes satiety (or the feeling of satisfaction), so it can help people especially when trying to lose weight.

Mitzi points out that women as well as men need more protein than most people realize. For instance, a woman in her mid-thirties on an average American diet probably gets about 55 to 60 grams of protein every day. Following the higher recommendations of the All-Pro Diet, that figure would jump to 95 to 100 grams of lean protein per day to help her stay satisfied in terms of her energy needs and to promote a more stable blood-sugar profile.

Of course, protein requirements do vary, especially among athletes, based on a person's body weight, training routine, and performance goals. Many athletes exceed the amount of protein that they need on a daily basis. However, Mitzi has also seen physically active individuals, including professional football players, not eat enough protein. Typically, these are the guys who skip meals. If they're eating only a couple of big meals a day, they're probably not getting enough protein.

My own target? Since I weigh in at 246 pounds and need between 0.7 and 0.9 gram of protein per pound, I shoot for at least 175 grams of protein per day. Just to give you an idea of what that means in terms of what I eat, my morning smoothie gives me about 26 grams, and a 7-ounce

Tony G.'s Nutrition Tip

Spinach is one of those nutrient-rich foods that's low in calories and high in nutrition. It is packed with powerful phytonutrients. In addition to these powerful compounds, it is loaded with powerful vitamins and antioxidants like vitamins A, C, E, K, B_1, and B_6, and minerals like calcium, potassium, and zinc. That's why I always like to add a handful of fresh baby spinach to any fruit smoothie to boost my nutrition. I highly recommend it!

serving of fish provides about 49 grams. So, on a daily basis, all I need from other sources is about 100 grams.

Calculating Your Own Daily Protein Requirements

As a starting point, it's fairly easy to figure out your protein needs based on your level of activity. Mitzi says the average active person wanting to gain muscle and lose fat—whether man or woman—should get 0.7 to 0.8 gram of protein per pound of body weight daily. The same range holds for strength athletes (gymnasts, weight lifters, etc.), though a professional football player might need to go as high as 0.9 gram per pound. For endurance athletes (long-distance runners, for instance), the needs are somewhat less—0.55 to 0.64 gram per pound.

Keep in mind, if you get too gung ho and end up with excessive protein intake, it may be stored as body fat and not converted to muscle because you are taking in too many calories. The daily protein requirements recommended by Mitzi are optimal for building muscle, which will help you burn fat throughout the day.

All-Pro Diet Protein Sources

Rule of thumb: 1 ounce of fish, poultry, or white meat provides about 7 grams of protein. Three ounces of these foods is about the size of a deck of cards.

Source	Amount	Protein (g)
Fish/Meats		
Chicken breast (no skin)	4 oz	30
Ground beef	4 oz	23
Pork tenderloin	3.5 oz	28
Salmon, grilled	3 oz	23
Snapper, broiled	3 oz	23
Tuna in water	3 oz	25
Egg		
Egg	1 large	6
Egg whites	2	7

Source	Amount	Protein (g)
Dairy/Nondairy Substitutes		
Almond milk	1 cup	1
Cottage cheese, 1%, organic	½ cup	14
Hard cheese	1 oz/1" cube	7
Hemp milk	1 cup	4
Milk, 1%, organic	1 cup	8
Rice milk	1 cup	1
Soy Products		
Edamame (soybeans)	1 cup	26
Tempeh	½ cup	19
Beans/Legumes		
Most beans	1 cup	14–15
Black-eyed peas	1 cup	10
Lentils	1 cup	18
Nuts/Seeds		
Almonds/peanuts	1 oz	6
Cashews	1 oz	4
Peanut butter	2 Tbsp	9
Sunflower seeds	1 oz	6
Walnuts	1 oz	7
Grains (cooked)		
Amaranth	1 cup	9
Barley	1 cup	4
Millet	1 cup	6
Oats	1 cup	6
Quinoa	1 cup	9
Rice, brown	1 cup	5

(continued on page 66)

All-Pro Diet Protein Sources (cont'd)

Source	Amount	Protein (g)
Nutritional Supplements		
Accelerade	1 cup	4
CherryPharm Recovery	1 cup	8
Plant-based protein powder (Tony Gonzalez All-Pro)	1 scoop	17
Hemp protein powder (Manitoba Harvest)	1 scoop	11
Rice protein powder (Rainbow Light)	1 scoop	15
Whey protein powder (Tony Gonzalez All-Pro)	1 scoop	25
Whey protein powder (Jay Robb)	1 scoop	25
Miscellaneous		
Pasta (whole wheat–dry)	¾ cup	7
CLIF Nectar energy bar	1 bar	3
LÄRABAR energy bar	1 bar	5
Raw Revolution energy bar	1 bar	7
PURE Bar energy bar	1 bar	6
PranaBar energy bar	1 bar	4
YouBar energy bar	1 bar	varies
Zing energy bar	1 bar	10

The goal for all of us is to stimulate muscle growth through optimal protein synthesis. Some nutritionists have suggested that vegetarians should slightly increase their protein intake (by about 10 percent) to make up for a lower digestibility of plant protein compared with animal protein. As for a maximum figure, many sports nutrition experts agree that there's no added benefit for athletes in going above 0.9 gram of protein per pound of body weight.

My own experience leads me to believe that athletes and anyone else who wants to build muscle should pay just as much attention to protein *timing* as protein *quantity*. Remember, just because some protein is good doesn't mean more is better, so avoid taking in excessive amounts. Mitzi says there's a lot of research that does, indeed, stress the importance of nutrient timing. What counts is not just *what* you eat but *when* you eat it. Consuming some protein before and after exercise has been shown to create an optimal anabolic environment for muscle growth. And, in my experience, that's what has worked best.

PROTEIN POWDERS—MY CHOICES

Protein powders can be an important part of an athlete's diet, especially if, like me, you have a limited intake of some of the common sources of protein. Powders allow you to boost protein intake without adding much in the area of carbs, fat, or extra calories. The majority of athletes do consume enough protein throughout the day, but a lot of it most likely comes from animal protein that is higher in saturated fats.

MITZI ADVISES . . .

When I'm talking with athletes about protein intake, I emphasize that it's a good idea to draw on many different sources. "Most research has shown that athletes require generous portions of lean, complete protein each day to perform at high levels and to build/maintain their muscle mass and their metabolism," notes John Berardi, PhD, an elite-level sports nutrition coach and faculty member at the University of Texas at Austin. "While some vegetable sources of protein are considered complete, most are not. Further, those vegetable sources of protein that are complete often contain very small amounts of protein relative to their carb and calorie contents. It's for this reason that intelligently designed plant-based diets usually contain a mixture of protein sources. Further, intelligent nutrition plans also focus on including protein-rich plant sources such as some fermented soy foods as well as supplemental proteins like rice protein, hemp protein, and pea protein."

If you follow Phase I and Phase II of the All-Pro Diet, you'll have ample opportunity to meet your protein requirements using many different sources.

Whey Protein Powder

Whey is a liquid byproduct of the cheese-making process. Whey powder—sold under many brand names—is the dried form. Whey protein is known as a fast protein, which means it is absorbed more quickly than other proteins. It has been assumed that using a fast protein instead of a slow protein (like some of the plant-based options) leads to greater gains in muscle-building. More research is needed in this area. In the meantime, Mitzi suggests that if you use whey instead of vegetable protein, look for a good whey protein powder from grass-fed cows. Also, read the label of any whey powder product to make sure that artificial sweeteners have not been added.

The whey protein in my diet now is found in my recovery drink and in any cheese I eat. I'm a believer in plant-based protein powders to ease my digestion. But feel free to substitute a whey protein powder if you prefer.

Plant-Based Protein Powders

Jon Hinds, the primarily vegan trainer I mentioned earlier, once came down to my football training camp in Wisconsin. He took me shopping to help me figure out what to eat and how to get enough protein. He advised me to consume a variety of pea, brown rice, and hemp protein. I also had the opportunity to meet and correspond with Dr. Colin Campbell, author of the great book *The China Study*. With more than 50 years of experience in nutritional studies, Dr. Campbell agreed that a variety of plant-based protein is the best way to meet your body's protein needs. I bought pea, brown rice, and hemp protein powder as well as flaxseeds and multivitamins to make sure I was meeting my nutritional goals. When I got to the checkout line, the total came up to a whopping $140. I was shocked to say the least, but if this was the price to pay for good health, I was willing to do it.

My original method was rather primitive—I would just put all the protein powders in a tub with the flaxseeds and mix them. I would then put one scoop into the smoothies I was making and drink it with the multivitamin. This routine worked well until I started thinking about how great it would be if there was a product that combined these three plant-based sources of protein with the flaxseed and multivitamin. I went to the store and couldn't find anything that came even close to what I was looking for.

Feeling deflated but not defeated, I then approached a reputable manufacturer who would be able to combine the brown rice, pea, and hemp protein plus flaxseed and multivitamin.

I was excited when I realized that not only were we able to manufacture this supplement, but it could be improved by scientifically formulating it in such a way as to provide optimum benefits using premium ingredients and adding natural flavoring to improve the taste.

So we set out to come up with the perfect protein supplement. It took a lot of time and hard work, but I'm happy to say we developed, in my opinion, not one but two excellent protein supplements: one made of 100 percent vegan proteins and one that is 100 percent whey protein using the highest-quality ingredients with whey protein isolate from grass-fed cows. The days and inconvenience of finding and combining all of these supplements, not to mention dropping $140 every 3 to 4 weeks, are over. I now have two great protein options with the capability of one-stop shopping at an affordable price (see the Resource Guide on page 227 for more information).

But it is also essential to *protect* what we build, therefore, I always make sure to include disease-fighting antioxidants in my diet to combat cellular damage from free radicals. We've all heard of açaí (ah-sigh-ee) by now, the nutritionally dense superfood that has made so many headlines for its powerful antioxidant qualities. Açaí is grown in the Amazon rainforest and yields açaí berries, which are packed with more antioxidants than blueberries. I have made a habit of consuming both an açaí juice and frozen açaí product as part of my daily regimen. However, most people like me who are very busy and must travel a lot cannot be tied down to a refrigerator or freezer and need another option.

So another healthy alternative is to consume high-quality açaí berries that are flash-frozen and then freeze-dried to maintain optimum nutritional content. With my busy schedule in mind, I developed an all-natural product that not only contains high-grade, freeze-dried açaí berries, but also two other powerful, antioxidant superfoods: goji berries and grapeseed extract. For an athlete, grapeseed extract is also beneficial because it is a natural anti-inflammatory. So, this is an easy way to provide the bodies of busy people with some additional antioxidants.

Hemp Protein Powder

Hemp protein powder is made from the cannabis plant, which of course is notorious as the source of marijuana. But hemp protein powder is just a food, with a negligible amount of THC (tetrahydrocannabinol, the hallucinogenic component in cannabis). It's completely legal, and the powder is totally natural. Hemp protein mixes well with other components of a morning protein drink and gives you some additional omega fatty acids.

You can purchase hemp protein powder online or at a health food store, and it's a great alternative to whey protein if you want a change.

Personally, I do not take creatine and have never felt that it really helped me when I did take it several years ago. It is definitely one of the most popular supplements among football players, and Mitzi has shared with me that the science does look pretty good to support its use by some athletes.

WHAT ABOUT SOY FOODS?

Most people realize that soy is a vegetarian source of protein, and I know a number of vegetarians especially who rely on this important source. In the All-Pro Diet, we do include some soy foods, but Mitzi isn't keen on a high-soy diet. There are a number of reasons.

In the nutrition world, there is currently quite a bit of controversy about soy. Soy naturally contains a large amount of toxins also known as *antinutrients*. It has a very high phytate level, which can block absorption of minerals. In addition, soy contains goitrogens, substances that depress thyroid function, and soybeans contain a clot-promoting substance called hemagglutinin. Soy is high in phytoestrogens, which can be good for you—but they can also have a bad effect (especially among women) related to cancer growth and menopause symptoms.

While soy has long been a significant component of the Japanese and Chinese diet, people don't realize that the majority of soy foods found in American grocery stores come from plants that have been genetically modified. In fact, Americans will find soy protein isolate and textured vegetable protein in many of their foods today that would be unfamiliar to Asian cultures. And soy is one of the foods most contaminated with pesticides.

Which soy foods are okay to eat? At the top of the list Mitzi puts fermented soy products such as miso, tempeh, and natto. She recommends having plain tofu occasionally (up to twice per month) and including some edamame in your diet. The bottom line is to avoid eating soy at every meal, and don't assume that you're eating healthily just because you pick up a supermarket product that advertises soy content. Many of the imitation meats made with soy found in supermarkets are anything but healthy. They are really just highly processed junk food. Instead, the All-Pro Diet includes soy as a condiment rather than as a staple of your diet.

KEEP YOUR SOLDIER COUNT STRONG: MINIMIZE SOY INTAKE

A study in the journal *Human Production* shows that a half serving of soy-based foods each day could lead to a decreased sperm count. The amount of soy consumption that resulted in a reduction in sperm count is equivalent to ½ cup of soymilk or a half serving of tofu every day. Possibly suggesting a hormonal link, the correlation was even stronger in overweight men. Overall, men with the highest soy intake had a significantly reduced sperm production compared with men not consuming soy products.

THE TRUTH ABOUT CARBS

It's a fact that carbohydrates will make you gain weight—as many people assume—but as Mitzi points out, that's *only* true if you eat too many carbs and calories. If you avoid carbs completely, you will definitely be lacking the necessary energy in your muscles to maximize your workouts.

Once Mitzi had a young NFL running back come see her because he had no energy. He told her his legs always felt "dead." He shared with her that his agent had hooked him up with a guy who put him on an extremely low carbohydrate diet. Now the player was frustrated because he said the coaches thought he was lazy. The truth was he really just didn't have any energy.

Mitzi told him about the All-Pro Diet, and he made the changes. He increased his carbs slowly and intelligently to keep his weight under control while also ramping up his energy.

Bottom line: You need to be sure you are eating plenty of high-quality carbs. They are the primary source of fuel for your muscles. If you severely restrict your carbohydrate intake, you'll feel the difference right away. Your muscles won't have the fuel they need to perform and recover optimally.

But also keep in mind the 17 All-Pro Diet Principles. Your carbohydrates should primarily come from fruits, vegetables, and whole grains instead of sugar-laden foods like sodas, chips, and refined carbs. You want your carbs to be nutrient-rich foods instead of empty calories or foods that make your pancreas work overtime trying to control your blood sugar.

While optimal carb intake varies, based on total caloric needs, the All-Pro Diet includes at least five servings of fruits and vegetables per day or about 2 cups of fruit and 2½ cups of vegetables per day. And remember to avoid added sugars. The All-Pro Diet wants to shift your diet away from added sugars like refined white sugar and high-fructose corn syrup, which, again, can actually increase your cravings for sweets. Too much sugar can impact energy levels and negatively impact energy and performance!

READING LABELS TO SPOT HIDDEN SUGARS

Added sugar and high-fructose corn syrup are hidden ingredients in many foods. You might think that a cup of strawberry yogurt is a healthy addition to your meal, but it may have the equivalent of 10 teaspoons of sugar. And a can of Mountain Dew has more than 11 teaspoons. With each teaspoon of sugar equal to 16 calories, that means you're getting more than 160 calories that have absolutely no nutritional value when you eat or drink foods like these.

When reading food labels, understand that many ingredients are just different forms of sugar. Here are some to look for: corn syrup, high-fructose corn syrup, fructose (fruit sugar), brown rice syrup, evaporated cane juice, dextrose, and fruit juice concentrate. Avoid foods when a sweetener is one of the first three ingredients listed on the package. (The label lists ingredients in order from most to least, so when one of these sweeteners is near the top of the list, it means the food is jam-packed with that ingredient.)

Of course, many fruits have a sweet taste, but that comes from natural sugars, which include lots of other important nutrients such as fiber and disease-fighting antioxidants. So it makes sense to opt for fruit instead of candy to satisfy a sugar craving.

ARTIFICIAL SWEETENERS

In the All-Pro Diet we encourage you to avoid artificial sweeteners, which can include aspartame (Equal and NutraSweet), saccharin (Sweet'N Low), and sucralose (Splenda). As noted when we were discussing the 17 All-Pro Diet Principles, these are all unhealthy, potentially toxic chemicals that pose risks to your health. With research suggesting that artificial sweeteners may contribute to carbohydrate cravings, we're pretty sure that people who get a lot of these sweeteners also tend to overeat. Ban them from your diet and make sure to read nutrition labels religiously, as many "light" or "no-calorie" drinks and foods contain artificial sweeteners. Some natural sweeteners that are okay by us are stevia, honey, and agave nectar. If you use a protein powder, remember to check the label and make sure it is free of artificial sweeteners—aim for either stevia or no sweetener. By choosing natural sweeteners, you won't be adding artificial, lab-created chemicals to your body.

THE FIBER BONUSES

One of the biggest improvements that I have made with my new diet is increasing my fiber intake. Fiber is important; it keeps everything running smoothly. Back when I was on my high-saturated-fat diet with lots of meat and dairy foods, I suffered for years from a poorly running gastrointestinal system. I don't have those problems any longer. Everything changed when I increased my intake of fruits, vegetables, beans, legumes, and whole grains. Consuming a high-fiber diet helps prevent constipation.

In addition, research has shown that soluble fiber can help reduce total blood cholesterol levels and therefore may reduce your risk of heart disease and some cancers. And there are other benefits as well. Including dietary fiber in your daily diet can help provide a feeling of fullness and add bulk to your diet. This may be helpful in controlling weight by making you feel satisfied sooner!

According to Mitzi, you also reduce your risk of diverticulosis when you're on a high-fiber diet. This is a serious health condition that occurs

MITZI ADVISES . . .

Tony mentioned a few foods that are high in fiber to include in your diet. Here's a comparison list to help you make choices:

1.0–1.5 G	1.6–2.0 G	2.1–3.0 G
Oatmeal (¾ cup)	Oat bran (⅓ cup)	Kidney beans (½ cup)
Broccoli (½ cup)	Carrots (½ cup)	Sweet peas (½ cup)
Sweet potatoes (½ medium)	Lentils (½ cup)	Prunes (5)
Apples (1 medium)	Oranges (1 medium)	Black-eyed peas (½ cup)

when a small bulging sac pushes outward from the colon wall. Someone with diverticulosis may have few or no symptoms, but when the sac (called a diverticulum) ruptures and becomes infected, the condition is called diverticulitis. If you're suffering from diverticulitis, you're likely to have a range of symptoms that characterize diverticular disease, including abdominal pain, abdominal tenderness, and fever. When bleeding originates from a diverticulum, it is called diverticular bleeding.

Soluble fiber can help lower cholesterol and blood-sugar levels. The soluble fiber absorbs water, forming a gel, and the gel traps cholesterol and sugar, preventing it from being absorbed from the intestine. It is then eliminated when you have a bowel movement. (Best sources of soluble fiber are oat bran, fruits, and dried beans.)

Insoluble fiber does not absorb water, but adds bulk to your stool, which aids in sweeping contents through your intestine. As a result, this type of fiber helps prevent constipation and colon cancer. (Sources of insoluble fiber include foods like wheat bran and whole wheat pasta.)

The American Dietetic Association recommends that every adult get 20 to 35 grams of soluble and insoluble fiber (collectively called dietary fiber) every day.

KITCHEN CONFIDENTIAL: HERE'S WHAT YOU'LL NEED

When I first started this diet, I wasn't cooking much. That's changed! Now I love to cook. If you tend to eat out a lot or you choose a lot of prepared food to avoid spending time in the kitchen, I think you might be surprised and pleased with how rewarding it can be to prepare healthy foods in your own kitchen. Not only will the meals be healthier, you'll also save money from eating out, ordering take-out, or buying high-priced prepared and packaged foods (it's always cheaper if you use fresh ingredients). Also, as much as I enjoy eating out, there's something special about cooking your own meal and then enjoying it with family and friends.

Before getting started, here are a few simple cooking supplies you'll need to have at the ready in your kitchen.

- Blender
- George Foreman grill
- Cutting boards
- High-quality knives
- Nonstick skillet
- High-quality cookware set with lids
- Stockpot
- Casserole dishes with lids
- Mixing bowls
- Nonstick bakeware
- Measuring cups and spoons
- Rubber spatulas

Cooking Oils

Extra-virgin olive oil is great on salads, but it's not for cooking. A cooking oil should never be heated past its smoke point—that's when the oil begins to decompose, which can generate harmful cancer-causing compounds. And since extra-virgin olive oil has a lower smoke point, it just isn't appropriate. Save it for dressings or adding to food that has already been cooked.

Regular olive oil is fine since it has a higher smoke point—but, again, you never want to heat it to the point where it starts smoking.

Macadamia nut oil, which is delicious, has a higher smoke point.

I also recommend coconut oil. It has acquired a reputation—unfairly, in my view—of being unhealthy, but it's not unless you use more than you need.

Almond oil is also very healthy and has a higher smoke point than both macadamia nut oil and coconut oil.

CHAPTER 5

THE ALL-PRO DIET PLAN

"LEAVING THE GAME PLAN IS A SIGN OF PANIC, AND PANIC IS NOT IN OUR GAME PLAN."

—Chuck Noll, Former Coach of the Pittsburgh Steelers

Okay, it's time to start a new lifestyle that will change your health. As I've mentioned, we've divided this program into two parts—Phase I and Phase II. During Phase I, we want you to focus on the 10 action items below. I'll list the foods that you should drop from your meals and snacks, which will get you into the habit of avoiding them permanently. During this first 2-week phase, you will be introduced to a new way of eating. You'll have the opportunity to try some new foods while letting go of some of the foods that are preventing you from being your best.

PHASE I ACTION ITEMS

1. Switch to whole grain products and eliminate refined-flour products from your diet. This means brown rice instead of white rice and whole grain bread instead of white bread.

2. Eat at least one plant-based meal each day.

3. Go food shopping at least two times per week (including the farmers' market and grocery store).

4. If you choose to consume red meat, limit it to no more than 4.5 ounces per week (18 ounces per month is the upper limit). Go with grass-finished beef.

5. When you have a meal, eat slowly and pay attention to whether your hunger is satisfied. When you reach the point where you're satisfied, stop eating! Don't eat to the point that you are full.

6. Eat at least one food that's a source of protein at every meal.

7. Every day, supplement with a daily multivitamin with minerals and omega-3 fish oil. (Consult with your physician first.)

8. Avoid eating after dinner if you are trying to lose weight.

9. Avoid all alcohol.

10. Take five highly processed foods out of your diet. (To help you get started, list those foods below.)

Personal Commitment List

The five foods I'm eliminating from my diet in Phase I are:

1. _____

2. _____

3. _____

4. _____

5. _____

To help you make this list, we've given you all the foods and ingredients you want to *permanently* avoid. In Phase I, begin with the first five that you listed above. In Phase II, go on to the next step, permanently removing the rest of these foods from your diet.

Foods and Ingredients to Permanently Avoid

- Fast food. (Like quarter pounders with cheese and french fries, for instance!)
- Refined flour products like white rice, pasta, breads, bagels, wraps, pancakes, and pitas. (You'll be switching to whole grain versions of these foods.)
- Hydrogenated and partially hydrogenated oils. (Many of the fried foods served in fast-food places use partially hydrogenated oils; these are also often found in bakery products and in regular peanut butter [choose natural]. Always read the food label and avoid the product if the ingredients list includes hydrogenated or partially hydrogenated oils.)
- Artificial sweeteners including sucralose (Splenda), aspartame (NutraSweet, Equal), acesulfame-K (Sunett), and saccharin (Sweet'N Low). (Some common food products that include these sweeteners are some yogurts, G2, Crystal Light, diet sodas, and many other drinks that advertise zero or low calories. So read the labels and look for the names of those sweeteners.)
- Soda, lemonade, fruit drinks, fruit punch, Kool-Aid, and sweet tea.
- Sodium nitrate and sodium nitrite. (Read the labels on deli meats and other foods that might contain these preservatives.)
- Canned fruits and vegetables (exception: canned tomatoes).
- Highly processed meats. (Read the labels to look for meats that have very minimal processing.)

MOVING FROM PHASE I TO PHASE II

If you feel like you need another week or two on Phase I before progressing to Phase II, that's fine. Take your time. During Phase II, you should aim to eat a diet even more focused on plant-based foods. This is where you'll essentially adapt every aspect of the All-Pro Diet, setting the pattern for a program that will last the rest of your life. Our goal is to allow you to experience a diet of nutrient-rich whole foods while eliminating foods that are unnecessary, unhealthy, and nutritionally useless.

PHASE II ACTION ITEMS

Here are the next steps to take as you make a full commitment to Phase II of the program.

1. Eat one to two plant-based meals per day.

2. Eat primarily plant-based snacks. (About one in four snacks can include animal products.)

3. Choose organic foods. If you include a small amount of dairy in your diet, make it a priority to *only* buy organic.

4. Try one to two new recipes per week. (The recipes in this book will get you started; once you're on the All-Pro Diet, keep looking for new recipes you can add so you don't get bored.)

5. Eat more slowly and avoid unconscious eating.

6. Find a farmers' market in your area and try to visit a local farm. (Visit www.localharvest.org to find local farmers' markets and family farms.)

7. Eliminate almost all highly processed foods from your diet. (In

---

A REASON TO SAY "CHEERS"

A recent study suggests nondrinkers who start to drink decrease their chances of developing heart disease. The findings in the journal *Alcoholism: Clinical and Experimental Research* showed a 38 percent reduction in the likelihood of a heart attack for middle-aged people. The typical recommended amounts are one to two drinks per day. In addition, the people who only consumed wine saw the biggest benefits. But don't think this is your pass to drink a lot all of the time. Those who drank five or more drinks a day were 30 percent more likely to experience heart attacks or strokes when compared to the one-drink-a-day people.

Phase I, I asked you to choose five foods to avoid as well as all highly processed meats. In Phase II, extend that list to include all highly processed foods.)

8. Eliminate all foods with artificial colors, flavors, and preservatives.

9. Limit alcohol intake to seven drinks per week.

10. Choose a primarily whole foods diet by eating foods with simple ingredients that are as close to nature as possible. A good rule of thumb: Buy foods with fewer ingredients, with the majority of your diet coming from single-ingredient foods.

ALL-PRO DIET FOOD MAKEOVERS

Take a look at this before-and-after list for ideas on how to make some easy changes in your diet immediately.

Before	After
Cakes, candies, cookies	Fresh fruit, dark chocolate (in moderation)
Cheese, cheese products	Organic 1% cottage cheese, guacamole
Potato chips	Popcorn, sweet potato chips, multigrain chips
Eggs	Free-range organic eggs with omega-3s
Fried fish	Baked or grilled fish
Fruit juice, fruit drinks (fruit juice with additives), soda	Water or green tea
Hot dogs, bacon, sausage	Pork tenderloin, pork chops
Commercial peanut butter	Natural/organic peanut butter, almond butter, cashew butter (only ingredients should be the type of nut and salt)
Salad dressing	Balsamic vinegar
White bread	Whole wheat bread, whole wheat pita, whole wheat wrap
White pasta	Whole wheat pasta
White rice	Brown rice, quinoa
Whole milk	Organic 1% milk, hemp milk, almond milk

GROCERY SHOPPING PLAN OF ACTION

I think we all understand that supermarkets are *not* in business to help you maintain a high-nutrition, low-calorie diet. When you walk into a supermarket, you enter a place where you have many food choices but no guide to steer you toward the foods that are best for your health. That's

RAISING ALL-PRO KIDS

As parents of young children, Mitzi and I are both just as passionate about helping to improve the nutrition of our country's children as we are about helping adults get healthier. American children are now facing shorter life spans because of the obesity epidemic. Thirty-two percent of children are now classified as either overweight or obese. One study suggests that 80 percent of children who are overweight from 10 to 15 years of age became obese adults. The term "adult-onset diabetes," once mostly seen in adults, is now called type 2 diabetes because so many young people now have the disease.

When you combine poor nutritional habits with lack of exercise, you get overweight children. With a generation of kids being raised on sodas, chips, french fries, and cheese-burgers instead of whole foods such as fish, whole grains, fresh fruits, and vegetables, the cards are stacked against them at an early age. Have you taken a look at the kids' menu at a restaurant lately? Typically, the choices are a hamburger with fries, a hot dog, chicken fingers, pepperoni pizza, or macaroni and cheese with a soda. Not exactly the picture of healthy nutrition. Kids today also prefer to play computer games and watch television, which takes away precious activity time.

Building a foundation of healthy nutrition habits from a young age is one of your most important jobs as a parent. Of course, setting an example as a healthy eater yourself is also very important. You need to eat a variety of foods and maintain a healthy weight if you want your children to do the same. Don't assume your kids won't like certain foods.

Here are nine ways to raise healthy kids:

1. **Introduce a variety of foods to your kids on a consistent basis, the earlier the better.** This is extremely important. It can take your child up to 20 times of trying a

why you need to use your own guidance mechanism—the All-Pro Diet—to help you make the best choices.

It's important to be aware of a few traps. When you see very large amounts of processed or packaged food advertised for a low price, beware! Manufactured food products are never a bargain. For the same

---

    new food until he or she actually enjoys it.

2. **Choose whole grains.** This includes bread, pasta, pancakes, tortillas, pita, cereal, crackers, and brown rice. It might not always be possible when eating out, but whole grains should be a no-brainer when making meals at home.

3. **Take your kids to the farmers' market weekly.** This is a great opportunity to have fun as a family while teaching them the importance of eating a whole foods diet. Let your kids pick their favorites!

4. **Avoid fast food.** It can certainly be tough when you have no groceries at home and you're on your way home from a soccer game, but try to limit the number of times you eat fast food in a week. Some kids are eating fast food twice a day. Research also shows that kids who attend schools closer to fast food are more likely to be obese.

5. **Get moving as a family.** Take walks, bike rides, or hike. Find local tennis courts, trails, or a track and get moving!

6. **Grow a garden.** When kids grow their own food, they are much more likely to eat it. This is a great way to teach them about the importance of eating fresh foods.

7. **Limit computer and video game time.**

8. **Encourage kids to play outside.** Kids stay inside too much, which limits activity. Encourage your kids to go outside and play—to go to the park, ride their bikes, ride their (mechanical) scooters, etc.

9. If you are trying to pick up a quick meal for your kid, stop by a local grocery store to buy some fresh fruits and vegetables along with a sandwich.

price, you could be getting fruits and vegetables that are much better stocked with nutritional content. If you take home big packages of processed food, there's a good chance you'll eat more and gain more weight. There's very little chance that you'll save anything in the long run, even if there are signs saying prices have been slashed.

Most importantly, before you head for the supermarket—before you even leave home—make a list that you're going to stick to. You need a plan of attack before you leave the house. Here are some guidelines:

1. Plan your menu a week ahead and put all of the necessary items on your grocery list. Don't stray from your list.

2. Never shop hungry. The temptation to buy an item that's not on your list is stronger when you're hungry.

3. Read food labels carefully. Look for high-fiber foods. Avoid foods with saturated fats and trans fats. Look for foods with short and simple ingredient lists with familiar words that are easy to pronounce.

4. Shop the perimeter. Start every shopping trip in the outer aisles of the store, purchasing the fresh food items on your list.

5. Aim to buy produce that is grown locally. It's more nutritious.

6. Choose organic whenever possible.

THE IMPACT ON YOUR GROCERY BILL

None of us can afford to be oblivious to the cost of food. When you move into Phases I and II of the All-Pro Diet, you'll begin to see some savings immediately. The longer you're on the plan, the more strategies you can develop to make sure your costs stay as low as possible while you're getting the best nutritional return on your money.

Meat is expensive. As soon as you begin limiting your meat servings to 18 ounces per month, you drastically slash your food costs. The foods that replace them at the heart of your diet—most notably beans, lentils, and quinoa—are extremely reasonable in price, especially if you buy in bulk.

Your All-Pro Diet breakfast foods are also cost-savers, especially if you buy them in bulk. Breakfast cereals are expensive food items. Instead of buying those high-priced, highly processed, and packaged items, all you need are rolled oats that are sold in large containers.

You're also saving big time when you stop spending money on sodas, sugary coffee drinks, or fruit drinks. To meet your fluid requirements, you don't have to buy bottled water. There are many kinds of reasonably priced water purifiers you can purchase to filter your home tap water.

Many kinds of organically grown produce are now available in big discount stores. These days, a store like Costco offers great organic products, and you can buy them in bulk. (During Mitzi's recent trip to a nearby Costco, some great finds included organic baby spinach, organic 1% milk, organic peanut butter, and whole wheat pasta.)

Other cost-saving tips:

1. Cook at home more often. This is a no-brainer; you can easily save money by simply reducing the number of meals you eat out, since eating in restaurants can get expensive very quickly.

2. When you do eat out, share an appetizer and an entree between two people. Most restaurants serve huge portions anyway.

3. Once again, avoid shopping on an empty stomach! When you're hungry, you're sure to buy more food than you really need.

4. Buy less food, make less food, and eat less food. The Okinawa population in Japan eats until they are 80 percent full and has one of the highest life expectancies in the world. Plus, you'll save money, which you'll need since you will be living longer!

5. Whenever possible, visit a farmers' market for your fruits and vegetables.

6. Avoid going into any store that sells "convenience foods" when you need a snack. Not only do these stores offer the wrong kinds of snacks, they often charge prices that are completely out of line with the value of what they offer.

7. Better yet, plan ahead for a snack attack and take a healthy snack with you when you leave the house, to work or anywhere else. Pack some fresh fruit, vegetables, or a clean energy bar.

8. Leftovers will save you money. If you only eat until you're satisfied and there's still food on your plate, save it for another day.

TOP 10 FOODS YOU MUST BUY AND TRY FOR THE ALL-PRO DIET

1. Quinoa

2. Chia seeds

3. Kale

4. Lentils

5. Avocados

6. Almond milk

THE GREEN TEA ADVANTAGE

There's a reason we recommend 2 cups of green tea a day in the All-Pro Diet. Findings from the *European Journal of Cardiovascular Prevention and Rehabilitation* showed that green tea improves blood flow and helps your arteries relax. The improvements are seen very quickly, within about 30 minutes. The beneficial properties in green tea are likely from the flavonoids. With heart disease being a leading cause of death, making the switch to green tea seems like an easy change for improved health.

7. Tart cherries (organic frozen or dried)

8. Green tea

9. Black beans

10. Natural nut butters (almond, cashew, peanut)

BUYING ORGANIC

As I have mentioned, I buy organic and locally whenever possible. It's not only a good way to reduce your exposure to pesticides but also a boon to the planet we live on. That means my first choice when shopping for produce is a local farmers' market that carries fruits and vegetables from local farms that maintain a pesticide-free environment. When I'm shopping for dairy, I always look for the "organic" label. And my small portions of meat come from grass-finished beef while my poultry is from free-range chickens.

With natural food sections expanding in mainstream grocery stores, these stores are another option, but you can often save money by shopping at farmers' markets. You also need to be aware that just because a food is labeled "organic," that doesn't necessarily mean it's healthy. Even if a package of cookies is labeled "organic," they are still cookies, which typically means they have a lot of calories, fat, and sugar. So be sure to use common sense if the word "organic" makes you automatically reach for a product.

There are still many discrepancies in food labeling policies. Sometimes smaller farms meet organic guidelines but can't afford the cost to become officially USDA-certified as organic. As Michael Pollan states in *In Defense of Food,* "Many, if not most, of the small farms that supply farmers' markets are organic in everything but name." If you're visiting a farmstand, just ask whether the farmer is an organic grower.

If you're not used to shopping and eating organically, here are two quick tips:

1. Keep in mind that eating nonorganic fruits and vegetables is more important than *not* eating fruits and vegetables at all. Again, use common sense here. The bottom line is if you're looking for organic produce and can't find it, it's better to eat nonorganic fruits and vegetables than deciding against eating fruits and vegetables at all.

2. Some pesticide residue can still be found in approximately 25 percent of organic produce (typically from pesticide drift from other farms). So all fruits and vegetables need to be washed before eating, whether they're organic or not.

The Dirty Dozen

If you choose organic whenever you're buying the "dirtiest" foods from the list below, the Environmental Working Group estimates you can cut your pesticide exposure by 90 percent. We call these foods "the dirty dozen" because they're highest in pesticides. To download your own pocket guide of the following information, visit www.foodnews.org.

1. Peaches
2. Apples

MITZI ADVISES . . .

If you tolerate dairy products, always choose organic. Not only do these products lack the antibiotics, hormones, and pesticides often found in nonorganic dairy products, in my opinion they taste better, too. If you're lactose intolerant, there are plenty of other options for you, such as hemp milk or almond milk. Although these milks aren't typically as high in protein, calcium, and vitamin D, you can make sure you get these important nutrients from other foods and possibly from supplements. In any case, on the All-Pro Diet, your consumption of animal products should be reduced.

3. Bell peppers

4. Celery

5. Nectarines

6. Strawberries

7. Cherries

8. Kale

9. Lettuce

10. Grapes (imported)

11. Carrots

12. Pears

The Clean Dozen

The following fruits and vegetables are the ones likely to be grown *without* a lot of pesticides. (I'd still advise buying organic when you're shopping for these foods, but you don't have to be quite as selective.)

1. Onions

2. Avocados

3. Sweet corn (frozen)

4. Pineapples

5. Mangoes

6. Asparagus

7. Sweet peas (frozen)

8. Kiwifruit

9. Cabbage

10. Eggplant

11. Papaya

12. Watermelon

(Source: Environmental Working Group)

KEEPING UP: JOIN THE SLOW FOOD MOVEMENT

There's a relatively new movement afoot called Slow Food that has recently been gaining momentum. This whole movement is doing great things for food and the environment. In a nutshell, those who subscribe to the Slow Food movement believe in eating food of high quality and excellent taste that comes from environmentally sustainable sources. The Slow Food movement is also about slowing down our fast-paced, fast-food lifestyle in order to enjoy life and have fun with family and friends.

The goals of the All-Pro Diet are very much in line with those of the Slow Food movement—and that's why I encourage you to find out more. Personally, I've become very interested in this movement, as has Mitzi, and I would say we're 100 percent behind "the Slow Food life," as proponents like to call it.

Want to start living the Slow Food life? Here's how to begin:

1. Shop at a local farmers' market (visit www.localharvest.org).

2. Join a Community Supported Agriculture (CSA) group. When you belong to a CSA group, you often pay a weekly amount, around $25, for a basket of different farm products such as fresh produce, eggs, poultry, and meat from local farms. There are many different types of CSA programs, so visit www.localharvest.org to investigate the options closest to you. There are now more than 2,200 CSA groups across the country.

3. Follow your food sources—find out where things come from.

4. Start your own garden in your kitchen. Mitzi does this! (For information, you can log on to www.aerogrow.com.)

5. Visit a local farm.

6. Read about food history.

7. Join a local Slow Food chapter or start your own!

For more information, visit www.slowfoodusa.com.

WANT TO HAVE 100 BIRTHDAYS?

If you would like to live to 100, take a look at two different towns where people live the longest. We can learn something from studying those populations who have long life expectancies. Just look at the people of Okinawa, Japan. Not only are they eating a diet similar to the All-Pro Diet, but they are also living a slow food lifestyle.

In Okinawa, people seem to age more slowly than the rest of us. They certainly enjoy more of a low-stress lifestyle, which has many similarities to the slow food life. They eat mostly a plant-based diet that includes fish, but some researchers think their most important habit for a longer life is their cultural tradition known as *hara hachi bu*, which means to eat until you're only 80 percent full. In other words, they don't stuff themselves. Eating a low-calorie diet seems to provide longevity to their population.

In Loma Linda, California, residents have the longest life expectancy of anyone in the United States. Loma Linda has a large Seventh Day Adventist population, and per the church's advice, many do not drink or smoke, and they eat a vegetarian diet. However, interestingly enough, even those who do not follow the church's rules live longer, so the spiritual connections derived from going to church might be powerful enough to provide greater longevity by reducing stress hormones.

ALL-PRO DIET FOODS TO EAT

Below you will find a list of foods that you can eat on the All-Pro Diet. You will see that you have lots of choices. Use this list as your grocery shopping list and also to keep lots of healthy options in your pantry, refrigerator, and freezer.

FRUITS

Apples
Apricots
Avocados
Bananas
Blackberries
Blueberries
Cantaloupe
Cherries
Coconut
Cranberries
Dates
Figs
Goji berries
Grapefruit
Grapes
Guava
Honeydew
Kiwifruit
Lemons
Limes
Mangoes
Nectarines
Oranges
Papaya
Peaches
Pears
Persimmons
Pineapples
Plums
Pomegranates
Prunes
Raisins
Raspberries
Strawberries
Watermelon
Dried fruit from above list (make sure it's sulfite-free)

VEGETABLES

Acorn squash
Artichokes
Arugula
Asparagus
Beets
Bok choy
Broccoli
Brussels sprouts
Butternut squash
Cabbage (green, Napa, red, savoy)
Carrots
Cauliflower
Celery
Collard greens
Corn
Cucumbers
Dandelion greens
Eggplant

MITZI ADVISES . . .

Eat lots of berries, as they are rich in vitamins and disease-fighting phytochemicals. Select fruits of varied colors and textures for fiber and nutrients. Aim to have a rainbow of colors on your plate.

Endive
Fennel
Garlic
Ginger, fresh
Green beans
Horseradish
Jicama
Kale
Leeks
Lettuce
Mushrooms
Okra
Onions
Parsnips
Peas
Peppers, bell (red, orange, green)
Peppers, chile (cayenne, jalapeño)
Pumpkin
Radicchio
Radishes
Rainbow chard
Red onions

Romaine lettuce
Rutabagas
Shallots
Snow peas
Spinach
Squash
Sweet potatoes
Swiss chard
Tomatoes
Turnip greens
Turnips
Water chestnuts
Watercress
Yellow squash
Zucchini

GRAINS

Amaranth
Barley
Brown rice
Buckwheat
Bulgur
Chia seeds
Corn tortillas

Couscous (whole wheat)
Durum wheat
Kamut
Millet
Oat bran
Oats (old-fashioned rolled oats and steel-cut)
Quinoa
Spelt
Teff
Wheat berries
Wheat bran
Whole wheat bread, pasta, pita, English muffins, etc.
Wild rice

CEREALS

Kashi—Go Lean, Good Friends, Heart to Heart, Organic Promise, Vive
Shredded wheat

FIGHT CANCER WITH BROCCOLI

Eating a little more broccoli each week just might help prevent prostate cancer in men. We know fruits and vegetables are cancer-fighters, but a specific compound in broccoli called sulforaphane might be the reason broccoli is able to turn on some genes that fight cancer and turn off those that promote it. (Prostate cancer is diagnosed in about 680,000 men each year worldwide.)

BEANS AND LEGUMES

Adzuki beans

Black beans

Black-eyed peas

Chickpeas

Green peas

Kidney beans

Lentils (brown, green, red)

Lima beans

Navy beans

Split peas

White beans (cannellini or great Northern)

NUTS, SEEDS, AND NUT BUTTERS

Almond butter

Almonds

Brazil nuts

Cashew butter

Cashews

Hazelnuts

Hempseeds

Macadamia nuts

Peanut butter

Peanuts

Pecans

Pine nuts

Pistachios

Pumpkin seeds

Sesame butter

Sesame seeds

Sunflower seeds

Tahini

Walnuts

Other nut and seed butters made from above list (natural only)

DAIRY

Butter/ghee, organic

Cheeses, organic (depends on source; look for natural, raw milk sources)

Chocolate milk, 1%, organic

Cottage cheese, 1%, organic

Cream cheese, reduced fat, organic

Goat's milk and cheese

Greek yogurt, low-fat, organic

Kefir, organic

Milk, 1%, organic

Plain yogurt, low-fat, organic (cow, sheep, goat)

Sheep's milk and cheese

Sour cream, light, organic

SOY PRODUCTS

Edamame (soybeans)

Fermented soy products (tempeh and miso)

"MY IDEA WAS TO DO EVERYTHING BETTER THAN ANYBODY ELSE EVER HAD. I CONCENTRATED ON EVERY ASPECT OF THE GAME."

—Willie Mays

Natto

Tofu (limit to twice monthly)

EGGS

Organic, cage-free, omega-3-enriched eggs

FATS AND OILS

Almond oil

Avocado oil

Coconut butter and oil

Extra-virgin olive oil

Flaxseed oil and flaxseeds

Hemp seed oil

Macadamia nut oil

Pumpkin seed oil

Sesame oil (unrefined, cold pressed, organic)

Walnut oil

FISH AND SEAFOOD

Cod

Crab

Flounder

Halibut, wild Alaskan

Herring

Lobster

Mackerel

Mahi mahi

Mussels

Oysters

Salmon, wild Alaskan

Sardines

Shrimp

Squid

Sturgeon

Tilapia, US

Trout

Tuna

Yellowtail

MEAT AND POULTRY

Free-range chicken breasts

Free-range turkey breasts

Grass-finished bison

Grass-finished filet mignon

Grass-finished ground beef

Grass-finished lamb

Grass-finished pork chop

Grass-finished pork tenderloin

Grass-finished venison

BEVERAGES, INCLUDING NONDAIRY MILKS

Almond milk

Açaí juice and smoothies from Sambazon

MITZI ADVISES . . .

Visit www.eatwild.com to find healthy sources of the meat, poultry, and game.

Coffee

Cranberry juice

Filtered water

Fresh vegetable
and fruit juices

Hemp milk

Pomegranate juice

Rice milk

Tart cherry juice

Tea (green, black,
white, and yerba
mate)

Wine (preferably red)

SWEETENERS

Agave nectar

Honey

**HERBS, SPICES,
AND CONDIMENTS**

All fresh/dried
herbs and spices;

some of the best are
listed below

Apple cider vinegar

Balsamic vinegar

Barbecue sauce

Basil

Black pepper

Broths, organic,
low-sodium
(vegetable and
chicken)

Cardamom

Cinnamon

Cloves

Cumin

Garlic

Ginger

Horseradish

Hot sauce

Ketchup, organic

Light mayonnaise
(Spectrum)

Mayonnaise
substitute
(Vegenaise)

Mustard

Oregano

Parsley

Pepper

Rosemary

Sage

Salsa

Sea salt

Soy sauce,
low-sodium

Thyme

Turmeric

OTHER

Chocolate, dark (at
least 70% cocoa)

ANTIAGING FOR THE HEART

According to a published study by *PLoS One*, resveratrol, a compound found in abundance in grapes and red wine, may have antiaging benefits for your heart. Another study showed that drinking red wine might also boost heart-healthy omega-3s in the body. The benefits have occurred when drinking in moderation, which is about one glass per day for women and one to two glasses per day for men.

YOUR UNWANTED FOODS LIST

When you start on the All-Pro Diet, you'll probably find a number of foods in your pantry and refrigerator that—how shall I put this?—you just won't need anymore. Should you throw them out? Give them away? Use them up?

The choice is yours. But whatever you do, make sure these foods are permanently eliminated from your kitchen as well as from your shopping list.

Fake meats

Hot dogs

ALL-PRO DIET SNACK IDEAS

1 whole wheat pita with 2 tablespoons hummus

30 pistachios

¼ cup walnuts

¼ cup almonds

10 baby carrots with 3 tablespoons hummus

Raw Revolution energy bar

LÄRABAR energy bar

CLIF Nectar bar

YouBar

Gnu Bar

PURE Bar

Prana Bar

Zing Bar

⅓ cup guacamole with 12 multigrain or sweet potato tortilla chips

AppleBoost energy snack tubes

1 orange

1 apple

1 cup berries

1 medium banana

1 cup fresh pineapple

2 cups watermelon

1 cup low-fat Greek yogurt

2 ounces salmon, venison, or beef jerky

½ tuna sandwich

1 hard-boiled egg

Cashew butter and honey sandwich (whole wheat bread)

Peanut butter and jelly sandwich (whole wheat bread)

Mini-smoothie (1 cup hemp milk with ¾ frozen banana)

Instant potatoes

Margarine

Pasteurized processed cheese food

Sausages

Soda

White pasta

White rice

CHAPTER 6

GETTING STARTED WITH THE ALL-PRO DIET MEAL PLAN

"YOU'RE EITHER IN OR YOU'RE OUT. THERE'S NO SUCH THING AS LIFE IN-BETWEEN."

—Pat Riley, NBA Coach

As a player, I know that if you want to learn any new skill, you have to start small, learn the basic steps first, and then build from there. Consider this chapter the first phase in developing a new skill set.

Here are some simple steps to meal planning and 7 days of meal plans to get you started on the All-Pro Diet. For each day, Mitzi has recommended menus for breakfast, lunch, dinner, and snacks. Needless to say, you can mix and match to suit your taste—but if you're just getting started, this 7-day plan is a great way to get into the groove and see what it's like.

The All-Pro Diet is not a one-size-fits-all diet. Everyone has their own unique calorie needs. Obviously, a 250-pound professional football player needs more calories than a 140-pound mom who goes to the gym 3 days a week. We never wanted to make this diet about counting calories, so if you are a smaller woman looking to lose weight, you probably want to decrease the portions slightly to cut out about 200 to 500 calories. You can skip an afternoon snack or cut back slightly throughout the day.

Rather than include all the recipes here, we've put them in the next chapter. Just refer to the page numbers in each menu.

In any menu that lists meat as an ingredient, you can substitute tempeh or occasionally seitan as alternatives. (However, most commercially prepared seitan is high in sodium, so a better option is to make your own.)

SIMPLE STEPS TO ALL-PRO MEAL PLANNING

1. Include a source of protein at every meal (refer to page 169 for daily protein goals).

2. Aim to eat at least 2 cups of fruit and 2½ cups of vegetables per day.

3. Eat a source of whole grains (many are listed below) at each meal with your protein. If you are trying to lose weight, you might need as little as 5 to 6 ounces per day.

One ounce = 1 slice of whole wheat bread or ½ cup brown rice, ½ cup whole wheat pasta, ½ whole wheat bun

For instance, 1½ cups whole wheat pasta = 3 ounces.

Here are some other whole grain options:

Amaranth	Whole grain cornmeal
Brown rice	Whole rye
Buckwheat	Whole wheat bread
Bulgur	Whole wheat crackers
Millet	Whole wheat pasta
Oatmeal	Whole wheat sandwich buns
Popcorn	and rolls
Quinoa	Whole wheat tortillas
Whole grain barley	Wild rice

PHASE I SAMPLE MEAL PLANS

DAY 1

BREAKFAST

Tony's Morning Power Smoothie (page 124)

SNACK

Slice of whole grain bread with 1 tablespoon peanut butter and 1 tablespoon agave nectar

Protein booster: 1 scoop protein powder (rice, hemp, or pea) mixed with ¾ cup milk (almond, hemp, or rice)

1 cup green tea

LUNCH

Lentil Soup with Apricots (page 139)

1 small whole wheat roll

SNACK

1 Raw Revolution energy bar

1 cup green tea

DINNER

Chicken Chili with White Beans (page 148)

Spinach Salad (page 141) with 2 tablespoons Balsamic Vinaigrette (page 158)

½ cup açaí sorbet

Totals: 2,089 calories, 121 g protein, 327 g carbohydrates, 63 g fat

If you work out today, make sure to choose a recovery drink from page 170. Drink it within 30 minutes of working out and include it as part of your total nutritional intake for the day.

DAY 2

BREAKFAST

1 cup cooked steel-cut oatmeal, made with water; add ½ cup blueberries and 1 scoop protein powder

1 cup green tea

SNACK

¼ cup raw almonds mixed with dried cranberries

1 ounce salmon jerky

LUNCH

Black Beans with Quinoa (page 151)

1 cup vanilla hemp milk

10 baby carrots

SNACK

1 Raw Revolution energy bar

1 cup green tea

DINNER

Whole Wheat Linguine with Shrimp (page 147)

Easy Asparagus (page 155)

1 ounce dark chocolate

Totals: 1,809 calories, 109 g protein, 228 g carbohydrates, 57 g fat

If you work out today, make sure to choose a recovery drink from page 170. Drink it within 30 minutes of working out and include it as part of your total nutritional intake for the day.

DAY 3

BREAKFAST

Mitzi's Berrylicious Smoothie (page 125)

SNACK

½ cup 1% organic cottage cheese

1 cup strawberries

1 cup green tea

LUNCH

Grilled salmon sandwich: 6 ounces salmon, grilled; whole wheat bun; 1 slice tomato; 1 tablespoon light mayo such as Spectrum Vegan Light Canola Mayo or ½ tablespoon Vegenaise

10.5-ounce bottle açaí juice

SNACK

40 pistachios

1 cup green tea

DINNER

Napa Cabbage White Bean Soup (page 138)

Quick Quinoa (page 155)

1 cup cooked carrots

1 ounce dark chocolate

Totals: 1,852 calories, 116 g protein, 223 g carbohydrates, 60 g fat

If you work out today, make sure to choose a recovery drink from page 170. Drink it within 30 minutes of working out and include it as part of your total nutritional intake for the day.

DAY 4

BREAKFAST

1¼ cups Kashi Vive cereal; mix 1 cup hemp milk with ½ scoop protein powder before pouring over cereal

SNACK

1 cup strawberries

1 cup green tea

LUNCH

Tuna salad sandwich: 6 ounces canned tuna; whole wheat pita; 1 slice tomato; 1 tablespoon light mayo such as Spectrum Vegan Light Canola Mayo or ½ tablespoon Vegenaise; 1 tablespoon pickle relish (optional)

2 cups watermelon

SNACK

¼ cup raw almonds

1 cup green tea

DINNER

Bison burger: 6-ounce grass-fed bison burger, grilled; whole wheat hamburger bun; 1 slice tomato; 1 tablespoon organic ketchup

Sweet Potato Fries (page 156)

½ cup orange sorbet

Totals: 1,817 calories, 112 g protein, 220 g carbohydrates, 62 g fat

If you work out today, make sure to choose a recovery drink from page 170. Drink it within 30 minutes of working out and include it as part of your total nutritional intake for the day.

DAY 5

BREAKFAST

Vegetable Scramble (page 135)

1 cup cantaloupe

1 cup green tea

SNACK

½ cup 1% organic cottage cheese with 1 cup fresh berries

1 cup green tea

LUNCH

Lentil and Brown Rice Salad (page 140)

1 apple

1 tablespoon any nut butter

SNACK

½ cup edamame

1 cup green tea

DINNER

Chicken fajitas: 6 ounces free-range boneless chicken, cooked; 1 whole wheat tortilla; ½ cup black beans; 2 tablespoons Guacamole (page 157); 2 tablespoons salsa

1 ounce baked tortilla chips

Guacamole

1 glass red wine

Totals: 1,941 calories, 144 g protein, 183 g carbohydrates, 68 g fat

If you work out today, make sure to choose a recovery drink from page 170. Drink it within 30 minutes of working out and include it as part of your total nutritional intake for the day.

DAY 6

BREAKFAST

Planet Earth Smoothie (page 133)

SNACK

40 pistachios

1 cup green tea

LUNCH

Black Bean Soup (page 137)

1 small whole wheat roll

10 baby carrots

Protein booster: 1 scoop hemp protein powder mixed with 1 cup hemp milk

SNACK

1 cup pineapple

1 cup green tea

DINNER

6 ounces grilled salmon

1 cup brown rice

1 cup Easy Steamed Spinach (page 153)

1 glass red wine

Totals: 1,884 calories, 110 g protein, 243 g carbohydrates, 48 g fat

If you work out today, make sure to choose a recovery drink from page 170. Drink it within 30 minutes of working out and include it as part of your total nutritional intake for the day.

DAY 7

BREAKFAST

Oatmeal Berry Bliss Smoothie (page 127)

SNACK

1 ounce salmon jerky

1 cup watermelon

1 cup green tea

LUNCH

Black Bean Soup (page 137)

1 small whole wheat roll

SNACK

1 LÄRABAR energy bar

1 cup green tea

DINNER

2 Fish Tacos (page 149)

1 cup steamed rainbow chard with dash of sea salt

Guacamole (page 157)

1 ounce baked tortilla chips

Totals: 1,786 calories, 117 g protein, 235 g carbohydrates, 38 g fat

If you work out today, make sure to choose a recovery drink from page 170. Drink it within 30 minutes of working out and include it as part of your total nutritional intake for the day.

PHASE II SAMPLE MEAL PLANS

(Note: Substitute tempeh or seitan as meat alternatives when desired.)

DAY 1

BREAKFAST

2 Banana Oatmeal Protein Pancakes (page 134) with 2 tablespoons agave nectar

SNACK

¼ cup cashews

1 cup green tea

LUNCH

Grilled chicken salad: 6 ounces grilled chicken; Spinach Salad (page 141); 2 tablespoons Balsamic Vinaigrette (page 158)

SNACK

Chocolate Nut Butter Smoothie (page 131)

DINNER

½ cup brown rice

1 cup black beans

2 cups steamed mixed vegetables

Totals: 2,087 calories, 144 g protein, 282 g carbohydrates, 54 g fat

If you work out today, make sure to choose a recovery drink from page 170. Drink it within 30 minutes of working out and include it as part of your total nutritional intake for the day.

DAY 2

BREAKFAST

   Coconut Dream Smoothie (page 126)

SNACK

   1 plum

   1 ounce salmon jerky

   1 cup green tea

LUNCH

   Quick Gazpacho (page 136)

   1 cup quinoa

   Protein booster: 1 scoop hemp protein powder mixed with 1 cup hemp milk

   1 apple

SNACK

   1 cup wild blueberries

   1 CLIF Nectar energy bar

   1 cup green tea

DINNER

   Lemon Honey Mahi Mahi (page 146)

   Easy Asparagus (page 155)

   1 cup brown rice

   1 glass red wine

   1 ounce dark chocolate

Totals: 1,929 calories, 102 g protein, 224 g carbohydrates, 64 g fat

If you work out today, make sure to choose a recovery drink from page 170. Drink it within 30 minutes of working out and include it as part of your total nutritional intake for the day.

DAY 3

BREAKFAST

Banana Berry Smoothie (page 128)

SNACK

1 cup steel-cut oatmeal, made with water; add ½ cup strawberries, 1 scoop protein powder, and 1 tablespoon agave nectar (optional)

1 cup green tea

LUNCH

6 ounces grilled chicken

½ cup whole wheat pasta

¼ cup marinara sauce

1 cup green tea

SNACK

10.5-ounce bottle açaí juice

DINNER

Vegetarian fajitas: 1 whole wheat tortilla; 1 cup black beans; ¼ cup brown rice; 2 tablespoons salsa; Guacamole (page 157)

1 cup fresh berries

1 glass red wine

Totals: 1,944 calories, 134 g protein, 248 g carbohydrates, 42 g fat

If you work out today, make sure to choose a recovery drink from page 170. Drink it within 30 minutes of working out and include it as part of your total nutritional intake for the day.

DAY 4

BREAKFAST

1 cup steel-cut oatmeal, made with water; add 1 scoop protein powder and 1 small handful of dried cranberries

1 cup green tea

SNACK

1 cup watermelon

LUNCH

Salmon salad sandwich: 6 ounces canned salmon; 1 slice whole wheat bread; 1 tablespoon light mayo such as Spectrum Vegan Light Canola Mayo or ½ tablespoon Vegenaise; 1 tablespoon pickle relish (optional)

1 cup green tea

1 orange

SNACK

Protein booster: 1 scoop hemp protein powder mixed with 1 cup hemp milk

DINNER

1 cup Kamut Salad (page 144)

1 cup broccoli

Spinach Salad (page 141) with 2 tablespoons Balsamic Vinaigrette (page 158)

Açaí Quinoa Dessert (page 160)

Totals: 1,700 calories, 111 g protein, 248 g carbohydrate, 62 g fat

If you work out today, make sure to choose a recovery drink from page 170. Drink it within 30 minutes of working out and include it as part of your total nutritional intake for the day.

DAY 5

BREAKFAST

1 cup Kashi Heart to Heart cereal; mix 1 cup hemp milk with 1 scoop protein powder before pouring over cereal

1 cup blackberries

SNACK

¼ cup raw almonds/dried tart cherries mixture

1 cup green tea

LUNCH

Chicken Curry Salad (page 142) added to a whole wheat pita

1 cup cantaloupe

SNACK

1 ounce salmon jerky

DINNER

Black Bean Soup (page 137)

1 small whole wheat roll

2 cups steamed dark leafy greens of your choice (spinach, kale, or rainbow chard)

1 glass red wine

Totals: 1,772 calories, 110 g protein, 239 g carbohydrates, 40 g fat

If you work out today, make sure to choose a recovery drink from page 170. Drink it within 30 minutes of working out and include it as part of your total nutritional intake for the day.

DAY 6

BREAKFAST

Banana Coconut Smoothie (page 132)

SNACK

1 cup fresh pineapple

1 cup green tea

LUNCH

Quick Quinoa (page 154)

1 cup beans of your choice

1 cup cooked greens (mustard, collard, kale, or rainbow chard) with dash of sea salt

SNACK

Waldorf Salad (page 143)

1 cup green tea

DINNER

Whole wheat pasta with meat sauce: 6 ounces grass-finished ground beef; ¾ cup marinara sauce; 1 cup whole wheat pasta

Easy Steamed Spinach (page 153)

1 ounce dark chocolate

Totals: 1,928 calories, 117 g protein, 244 g carbohydrates, 61 g fat

If you work out today, make sure to choose a recovery drink from page 170. Drink it within 30 minutes of working out and include it as part of your total nutritional intake for the day.

DAY 7

BREAKFAST

1 cup steel-cut oatmeal, made with water; add ½ scoop protein powder, 1 tablespoon agave nectar, and 1 small handful of raisins

1 cup blueberries

SNACK

40 pistachios

1 cup green tea

LUNCH

Black Bean Burger (page 150) on 1 whole wheat bun

10 baby carrots

SNACK

½ portion Banana Berry Smoothie (page 128)

1 cup green tea

DINNER

Cilantro Grilled Salmon (page 145)

Baby Bok Choy with Cashews (page 152)

1 cup brown rice

Berry Crumble (page 159)

Totals: 1,941 calories, 105 g protein, 269 g carbohydrates, 57 g fat

If you work out today, make sure to choose a recovery drink from page 170. Drink it within 30 minutes of working out and include it as part of your total nutritional intake for the day.

ALL-PRO ON-THE-GO

In addition to these meal plans, you'll need some strategies to help you stay on the All-Pro Diet when you're traveling or eating out.

I definitely don't eat out as much as I did before my new diet, since I enjoy cooking more now. But I still relish going to a good restaurant with family and friends. When I do dine out, it's no problem if I go to one of those favorite restaurants that I've scoped out beforehand. But even if I'm going to a place I've never been, I can figure out how to eat healthfully and in keeping with the All-Pro Diet. For example, if I go to an Italian restaurant, I'll typically order angel hair pasta with salmon, black olives, artichokes, mushrooms, and eggplant. And I'll eat my Italian bread with olive oil but never butter. Unfortunately, most restaurants don't offer whole wheat pasta or many of the other whole grains that we recommend in the All-Pro Diet. You have some flexibility when eating out; use common sense. Just watch your portion sizes!

Since I also travel a lot, I have to make lots of food choices in different environments. Some airports are easier to grab quick, healthy meals in than others. Avoid the fast-food options and look for some sort of restaurant that will make foods to order. For example, at a Mexican restaurant you could have grilled chicken and black beans with a little salsa. Or, you might choose some salmon with a side of vegetables. You could also have a sandwich on whole wheat bread with chicken or turkey.

Obviously, most of the chicken and turkey served in an airport is not free-range, but you have to eat, so don't be overly rigid or avoid eating. I would advise you to travel with some easy snacks like almonds and dried cherries or cranberries and keep some energy bars on hand in case you're in a hurry and get stuck without any healthful food choices.

Here are some nutritious tips for dining out and traveling. Look for the key words in the chart on page 116 to help you make smart and healthy choices when eating out:

Look for . . .	Avoid . . .
These words mean little or no butter or oil and great flavors.	These words mean added fat and rich dishes you'll want to steer clear of.
Au jus	Au gratin
Au vin	Basted
Baked	Batter-dipped
Broiled	Béarnaise sauce
Consommé	Béchamel sauce
Dry rub	Bordelaise sauce
Fresh	Breaded
Herb/herb-crusted	Buttery
Light	Casserole
Light pan sauce	Cheesy
Loin (lean cut of beef)	Creamy
Marinara	Crispy
Marinated	En croûte
Poached	Escaloped
Red sauce	Fried
Roasted	Hollandaise
Round (lean cut of beef)	In gravy
Steamed	Rich
Stir-fried in broth	Sautéed
Tomato-based	Smothered
Whole grain	Stir-fried in oil
Yogurt sauces	Stuffed

Even if some of your meals are eaten away from home, you can still make better choices. These tips will help you make the best choices at every restaurant.

- Visit the restaurant's menu online to get an idea of what you might order.
- Contact the restaurant in advance to find out if special preparation requests will be honored.
- In the restaurant, be assertive but very gracious about what you want.
- If you are choosing a meat, always choose an entrée that has the word *loin* in it, to get the leaner cut of meat.
- If you want dessert, share it and pick those with less fat and sugar, such as fresh fruit and sorbets.

Ask your waiter to:

- Clarify how a menu item is prepared.
- Prepare dishes without added salt or monosodium glutamate (MSG).
- Prepare dishes using cooking oils free of trans fats.
- Remove extra chips, rolls, and butter from the table.
- Suggest foods that are steamed, broiled, roasted, grilled, or poached.
- Serve salad dressings, sauces, and gravies on the side.
- Prepare dishes without added oil, butter, or margarine.
- Hold the mayonnaise on sandwiches; use mustard or a slice of avocado instead.
- Substitute baked potatoes, french fries, or onion rings with steamed vegetables.
- Steam your vegetables without sauce.
- Provide fat-free or low-fat milk with your coffee instead of cream.
- Serve whole grains like brown rice, wild rice, whole wheat bread, and pasta when available.
- Grill or bake a fish entrée.
- Wrap extra food to go. (Restaurants tend to serve large portions, so try to leave some food on your plate to avoid overeating.)

Fueling Yourself in Transit

When you're flying, it's important to stay well hydrated! This will help you feel more energized and alert. Consider purchasing a large bottle of water (inside the security checkpoint, of course) before takeoff, and make it a goal to finish that bottle before you land—and don't forget to continue drinking water after your flight!

Also as I mentioned, consider taking along some snacks for the flight. This will help you sustain energy and prevent overeating after the flight. Healthy snacks that are easy to carry on board include fresh fruit and energy bars like PURE Bar, Zing, Gnu, Prana, Raw Revolution, LÄRABAR, or CLIF Nectar (these all have fruit and nuts but no artificial ingredients). Or take along a sandwich on whole grain bread—peanut butter and jelly, cashew butter and honey, tuna, or chicken breast.

And if you're staying in a hotel, consider these healthy options when you get room service or eat in the dining room:

BREAKFAST
- Oatmeal with 1 scoop of your own protein powder and fresh berries
- Egg-white omelet with vegetables and fresh berries
- Fresh fruit smoothie; add your own protein powder

LUNCH/DINNER
- Fresh greens topped with salmon or chicken and balsamic dressing
- Grilled chicken breast sandwich with side salad
- Grilled fish with wild rice and steamed vegetables; sorbet for dessert

WATCH WHAT YOU DRINK

A lot of athletes (and others as well!) just don't realize how many calories they drink. These calories typically come from juice, alcohol, sodas, lemonade, fruit punch, sweet tea, and specialty coffee drinks loaded with extra calories. Mitzi had a client who was an NBA player and needed to lose some weight, but his activity was limited due to an injury. The coaches were concerned he would gain more weight during rehab, so they asked Mitzi to meet with him. After reviewing his diet, she found that he was drinking nearly 2,000 calories of grape juice every day! Once he cut out the juice, he became much leaner (even with his lower activity level). At one point, Mitzi posted a sign in the cafeteria where we players ate that read, "You can gain 22 pounds a year (80,300 calories!) by drinking only one extra 16-ounce glass of orange juice (220 calories) every day!" I didn't believe it at first and asked Mitzi about it, but you can't argue with the math. And if weight is an issue (as it is for many players, as well as the rest of us), a very simple step to reduce your calorie intake is to avoid drinking juice.

In the All-Pro Diet, of course, we don't advocate the use of artificial sweeteners, so read labels and avoid diet sodas and other artificially sweetened drinks like Crystal Light. Aim to avoid foods with aspartame, sucralose, and acesulfame-K, which are frequently found in "light" or "nonfat" yogurts as well. Remember, we want you to put foods into your body that are as close to nature as possible!

If you are happy with your current weight, avoid all high-sugar drinks like Kool-Aid and soda. You can drink 100 percent fruit juice in moderation; my favorites are those that provide additional benefits like the powerful antioxidants and healthy omegas in açaí juice or the phenolic compounds in tart cherry juice. However, keep in mind that you should avoid drinking any juice in large volumes.

Here's a comparison guide to help you make smart choices about beverages.

Calorie Content of Common Beverages

100% Fruit Juices:

Apple (8 oz)	117
Carrot (8 oz)	98
Cherry (8 oz)	130
Cranberry (8 oz)	137
Grapefruit (8 oz)	101
Orange (8 oz)	112

Hot Beverages:

Brewed coffee—decaf or regular (6 oz)	4
Green tea	0
Starbucks Caffè Americano (16 oz)	15
Starbucks Caffè Latte with fat-free milk (16 oz)	130
Starbucks Caffè Latte with whole milk (16 oz)	220
Starbucks Caffè Vanilla Frappuccino with whipped cream (16 oz)	430
Starbucks Hot Chocolate with fat-free milk and no whipped cream (16 oz)	240
Starbucks Hot Chocolate with whole milk and whipped cream (16 oz)	400
Tazo Chai Frappuccino Blended Crème with whipped cream	440
Tea, black (6 oz)	2

Miscellaneous Drinks:

Fruit punch (8 oz)	120
Hemp milk—vanilla (8 oz)	130
Lemonade (8 oz)	96
Organic 1% milk (8 oz)	100
Organic whole milk (8 oz)	150
Red Bull Energy Drink (8 oz)	108
Sambazon Açaí Juice (8 oz)	110
Sambazon Açaí Smoothie (8 oz)	140
Water	0

Specialty Waters:	
LifeWater (20 oz)	125
VitaminWater (20 oz)	125
Sports Drinks:	
Accelerade (20 oz)	233
Cytomax (20 oz)	200
Gatorade (20 oz)	125
Powerade (20 oz)	75
Sodas:	
Cola (12 oz)	143
Lemon-lime (12 oz)	147
Mountain Dew (12 oz)	165
Orange (12 oz)	180
Root beer (12 oz)	152
Sugar-Free Drinks (contain artificial sweeteners):	
Crystal Light	0
Diet Coke	0

IS YOUR ALCOHOL CONSUMPTION SABOTAGING YOUR ATTEMPTS TO LOSE FAT?

The bottom line is to stay away from alcohol as much as possible when you are trying to lose body fat. As I've mentioned before, alcohol is high in calories, low in nutritional value, and while you're drinking it, your liver is so busy absorbing it that it delays the fat-burning process, leading to greater fat storage.

Here's what those alcohol calories look like:

Bud Light (12 oz)	110
Budweiser (12 oz)	150
Coors Light (12 oz)	102

(continued)

Corona (12 oz)	148
Gin, rum, vodka, whiskey (1½ oz, 80 proof)	100
Gin, rum, vodka, whiskey (1½ oz, 100 proof)	124
Miller Light (12 oz)	96
Rum and Coke (4½ oz)	150
Wine, red or white (4 oz)	103

ALL-PRO ALCOHOL RULES

Okay, so you decide to have a drink at the bar anyway. What are the best ways to keep your calorie gain to a minimum?

First of all, obviously, avoid binge drinking. As you can see from the table above, a six-pack of regular beer weighs in around 900 calories, and even if you drink light beer, you'll have to burn about 600 extra calories. To burn that number of calories, you'd better plan on running 1½ hours *straight*.

If you're just having one drink—and that's it—here's what I advise:

1. Avoid salty bar snacks. Bar owners are smart. They know salty snacks make you want to drink more alcohol and eat more chicken wings and fries. When drinking, try to keep healthy options available since your inhibitions are weakened.

2. Always drink a glass of water along with your alcohol. Water can provide a feeling of fullness while keeping you hydrated.

3. Choose drinks with a lower number of calories but a higher content of alcohol—like wine.

4. If you're going to have beer, choose light beer.

Remember . . . on the All-Pro Diet, the rule is *no alcohol* in Phase I and a limit of *7 drinks per week* in Phase II.

CHAPTER 7

ALL-PRO RECIPES

"WHAT WE DO TODAY, RIGHT NOW, WILL HAVE AN ACCUMULATED EFFECT ON ALL OUR TOMORROWS."

—Alexandra Stoddard, Author and Philosopher

Now it's time for the fun part of the journey. I used to define my ability to cook by how many steaks I could throw on the grill. I've come a long way since I first reduced my dairy and red meat consumption. I love to cook now; here are some of my favorite recipes that Mitzi has created, which will allow you to take full advantage of what the All-Pro Diet has to offer. I promise that you don't need any cooking skills to prepare these meals. All you need is a commitment to do something good for your body and for your mind.

The payoff from changing your diet is immediate. Not only will you have much more energy, but you'll be able to think more clearly and process information more efficiently. Your brain is impacted by your diet. These clean recipes will help you mentally, physically, and spiritually—that's what I mean by a *whole foods diet*.

RECOVERY DRINKS

TONY'S MORNING POWER SMOOTHIE

Makes 1 serving (18 ounces)

¾ cup hemp milk

½ Sambazon Açaí Smoothie Pack

¼ cup coconut nectar

1 scoop protein powder blend of hemp, pea, rice, soy protein (I mix all these protein powders together)

3 fresh strawberries (can also be frozen)

1 handful blueberries

1 handful frozen cherries

3 baby carrots

1 large handful fresh baby spinach

Blend well and enjoy!

Per Serving: 403 calories, 26 g protein, 68 g carbohydrates, 8 g fat

MITZI'S BERRYLICIOUS SMOOTHIE

Makes 1 serving (16 ounces)

1 cup hemp milk or organic 1% cow's milk

1 cup frozen mixed berries

1 scoop protein powder (hemp or whey)

1 large handful fresh baby spinach

Blend well and enjoy!

Per Serving: 282 calories, 29 g protein, 41 g carbohydrates, 3 g fat

COCONUT DREAM SMOOTHIE

Makes 1 serving (8 ounces)

½ cup vanilla hemp milk

½ cup chilled light coconut milk

1 scoop protein powder (hemp, pea, rice, or whey)

1 frozen banana, slightly thawed

Blend well and enjoy!

Per Serving: 374 calories, 18 g protein, 46 g carbohydrates, 16 g fat

MITZI'S SMOOTHIE TIP

When freezing bananas for smoothies, peel them first and then put 3 or 4 in a freezer bag.

OATMEAL BERRY BLISS SMOOTHIE

Makes 1 serving (16 ounces)

1 cup hemp milk

1 cup frozen mixed berries

1 scoop protein powder (hemp, pea, rice, or whey)

¼ cup rolled oats

Blend well and enjoy!

Per Serving: 370 calories, 27 g protein, 52 g carbohydrates, 5 g fat

BANANA BERRY SMOOTHIE

Makes 1 serving (16 ounces)

1 cup milk (hemp, almond, rice, or organic 1% cow's)

½ cup frozen mixed berries

1 frozen banana, slightly thawed (can use banana at room temperature)

1 scoop protein powder (hemp, pea, rice, or whey)

2 tablespoons ground flaxseeds

Blend well and enjoy!

Per Serving: 412 calories, 32 g protein, 55 g carbohydrates, 9 g fat

PEACH MANGO SMOOTHIE

Makes 1 serving (16 ounces)

1 fresh mango, peeled and diced

½ cup frozen peaches

½ cup coconut juice

¾ cup hemp milk

2 teaspoons vanilla

1 scoop protein powder (hemp, pea, rice, or whey)

Blend well and enjoy!

Per Serving: 380 calories, 23 g protein, 59 g carbohydrates, 4 g fat

CHOCOLATE BANANA SMOOTHIE

Makes 1 serving (8 ounces)

1 cup milk (hemp, almond, rice, or organic 1% cow's)

1 banana, frozen but slightly thawed

1 scoop chocolate protein powder (hemp, pea, rice, whey)

Blend well and enjoy!

Per Serving: 345 calories, 23 g protein, 55 g carbohydrates, 5 g fat

CHOCOLATE NUT BUTTER SMOOTHIE

Makes 1 serving (18 ounces)

1 cup milk (hemp, almond, rice, or organic 1% cow's)

1 tablespoon any natural nut butter

1 scoop chocolate protein powder (hemp, pea, rice, whey)

6 ice cubes

Blend well and enjoy!

Per Serving: 312 calories, 30 g protein, 24 g carbohydrates, 11 g fat

BANANA COCONUT SMOOTHIE

Makes 1 serving (12 ounces)

1 cup milk (hemp, almond, rice, or organic 1% cow's)

1 frozen banana, slightly thawed

1 scoop protein powder (hemp, pea, rice, or whey)

2 tablespoons unsweetened coconut

Blend well and enjoy!

Per Serving: 395 calories, 30 g protein, 46 g carbohydrates, 13 g fat

PLANET EARTH SMOOTHIE

Makes 1 serving (10 ounces)

1 cup hemp milk

1 large handful baby spinach

1 frozen banana, slightly thawed

1 scoop hemp protein powder

Blend well and enjoy!

Per Serving: 395 calories, 22 g protein, 65 g carbohydrates, 9 g fat

BREAKFAST

BANANA OATMEAL PROTEIN PANCAKES

Makes 2 servings (2 pancakes per serving)

½ cup whole wheat flour

½ cup rolled oats

1 tablespoon raw honey

1 teaspoon baking powder

1 banana

1 scoop vanilla protein powder

¼ cup wheat germ

¾ cup vanilla hemp milk

1 teaspoon vanilla

1. Put the flour, oats, honey, baking powder, banana, protein powder, wheat germ, milk, and vanilla in a blender, and puree until smooth.
2. Pour about ¼ cup for each pancake on a lightly oiled griddle or skillet and brown on both sides.

Serve with fresh berries and 1 tablespoon agave nectar.

Per Serving (without topping): 393 calories, 22 g protein, 68 g carbohydrates, 5 g fat

VEGETABLE SCRAMBLE

Makes 4 servings

2 whole cage-free eggs + 6 whites of cage-free eggs

⅓ cup organic 1% milk or hemp milk

1¼ cups vegetables of your choice (such as fresh spinach, bell peppers, tomatoes, onions)

Salt

Pepper

1. Beat together the whole eggs, egg whites, and milk, and cook in a nonstick skillet on medium heat.
2. Sauté the vegetables separately and add them to the egg mixture slightly before the eggs are completely cooked. Salt and pepper to taste.

Per Serving: 293 calories, 32 g protein, 14 g carbohydrates, 12 g fat

SOUPS
QUICK GAZPACHO

Makes 6 servings

1 can (28 ounces) diced tomatoes
½ cup tomato juice
2 tablespoons extra-virgin olive oil
1 large cucumber, chopped
1 yellow bell pepper, chopped
1 small onion, diced
3 cloves garlic, chopped
2 tablespoons fresh lime juice
2 tablespoons fresh basil, chopped
2 teaspoons sea salt
1 teaspoon freshly ground black pepper

1. Combine half the can of tomatoes with the tomato juice, oil, cucumber, bell pepper, onion, garlic, lime juice, basil, salt, and pepper in a blender or food processor and puree to combine, but leave some texture.
2. Put in a bowl along with the remainder of the tomatoes. Refrigerate at least 2 hours prior to serving (you can refrigerate overnight).

Per Serving: 80 calories, 2 g protein, 13 g carbohydrates, 2 g fat

BLACK BEAN SOUP

Makes 6 servings

2 teaspoons macadamia nut oil

1 large onion, chopped

5 cloves garlic, chopped

1 tablespoon chili powder

1 tablespoon ground cumin

2 cups vegetable broth or reduced-sodium chicken broth

4 cans (15 ounces each) black beans

1 cup frozen corn

1 can (15 ounces) crushed tomatoes

1. Heat the oil in a large stockpot. Sauté the onion and garlic for about 4 minutes. Add the chili powder and cumin, and cook for 1 minute. Add the broth, 2 cans of black beans, and frozen corn. Bring to a boil.
2. In a blender, add the remaining 2 cans of beans and the tomatoes, with juice. Blend until smooth. Add to the soup, reduce heat, and simmer for 15 to 20 minutes.

Variation: Add baby carrots to the onion and garlic mixture for an extra boost of beta-carotene!

Per Serving: 300 calories, 17 g protein, 52 g carbohydrates, 4 g fat

NAPA CABBAGE WHITE BEAN SOUP

Makes 6 servings

2 teaspoons macadamia nut oil

1 large yellow onion, chopped

3 cloves garlic, minced

5 cups vegetable broth or reduced-sodium chicken broth

1 head of Napa cabbage

1 can (15 ounces) black-eyed peas

1 can (15 ounces) chickpeas

Sea salt

Freshly ground black pepper

1. Heat the oil in a large stockpot. Sauté the onion and garlic until soft.
2. Add the broth and simmer for 10 minutes.
3. Cut the base off the cabbage and peel off the leaves. Wash the leaves thoroughly and tear into bite-sized pieces. Add the cabbage to the pot and bring to a boil. Reduce heat and simmer for an additional 15 minutes. Add the black-eyed peas and chickpeas. Simmer until the cabbage is completely cooked. Season with salt and pepper.

Variations: Substitute the Napa cabbage with kale or collard greens. Add 1 cup baby carrots.

Per Serving: 228 calories, 15 g protein, 36 g carbohydrates, 4 g fat

LENTIL SOUP WITH APRICOTS

Makes 6 servings

2 teaspoons macadamia nut oil

1 small onion, chopped

2 cloves garlic, minced

1½ cups red lentils

¼ cup dried apricots

2 cans (14 ounces each) vegetable broth or reduced-sodium chicken broth

1 can (14 ounces) diced tomatoes with juice

1 teaspoon ground cumin

½ teaspoon dried thyme

Sea salt

Freshly ground black pepper

2 tablespoons fresh lemon juice

1. Heat the oil in a large stockpot. Sauté the onion and garlic until soft. Add the lentils, apricots, and broth and bring to a boil. Reduce heat and simmer for about 20 minutes.
2. Add the tomatoes and juice, cumin, thyme, sea salt, and pepper. Simmer for 10 minutes.
3. Add the lemon juice, and puree half the soup in a blender, then add it back to the pot. Mix together and serve.

Per Serving: 227 calories, 14 g protein, 39 g carbohydrates, 3 g fat

SALADS
LENTIL AND BROWN RICE SALAD

Makes 6 servings

½ cup uncooked brown rice

1 cup vegetable broth or reduced-sodium chicken broth

1 cup cooked lentils

1 medium tomato, diced

2 tablespoons red wine vinegar

1 tablespoon extra-virgin olive oil

2 cloves garlic, minced

2 teaspoons lemon juice

2 teaspoons Dijon mustard

Sea salt

1. Bring the rice and broth to a boil over medium heat in a saucepan. Cover and simmer for 35 minutes, or until rice is tender.
2. Combine the cooked rice, lentils, and tomato in a bowl. Combine the vinegar, oil, garlic, lemon juice, mustard, and salt in a small bowl and pour over the rice mixture, then toss to coat. Cover and refrigerate for 60 minutes.

Per Serving: 125 calories, 5 g protein, 21 g carbohydrates, 3 g fat

SPINACH SALAD

8 cups fresh baby spinach

½ cup walnuts

⅓ cup dried cranberries

¼ cup Gorgonzola cheese

Toss the spinach, walnuts, cranberries, and cheese together, and add Balsamic Vinaigrette (page 158).

Variation: Add 6 ounces grilled chicken breast or salmon per serving.

Per Serving (without chicken or salmon): 214 calories, 7 g protein, 37 g carbohydrates, 13 g fat

CHICKEN CURRY SALAD

Makes 6 servings

3 cooked skinless, boneless free-range chicken breasts, cubed

2 ribs celery, diced

1 cup green seedless grapes

½ cup almonds, slivered

⅓ cup grapeseed oil vegenaise or light mayo such as Spectrum Light Mayo

Sea salt

Stir together the chicken, celery, grapes, almonds, vegenaise or mayo, and salt in a medium bowl. Serve as is or with one-half whole wheat pita.

Per Serving: 293 calories, 29 g protein, 7 g carbohydrates, 16 g fat

WALDORF SALAD

Makes 8 servings

4 Granny Smith apples, diced

3 ribs celery, diced

2 cups red grapes

¾ cup walnuts, chopped

⅓ cup grapeseed oil vegenaise or light mayo such as Spectrum Light Mayo

Stir together the apples, celery, grapes, walnuts, and vegenaise or mayo in a medium bowl.

Per Serving: 200 calories, 2 g protein, 19 g carbohydrates, 14 g fat

KAMUT SALAD

1 cup kamut

3½ cups water

1 tablespoon extra-virgin olive oil

¼ cup red wine vinegar

¼ cup onion (1 small onion)

½ cup red bell pepper (1 small pepper)

1 large tomato, diced

¼ cup almonds, slivered

¼ cup dried tart cherries

1 cup cooked beans

4 tablespoons fresh basil

1. Cook the kamut and water in a covered saucepan over medium heat for 40 to 50 minutes, or until softened. Let cool.
2. In a medium bowl, combine the kamut, oil, vinegar, onion, bell pepper, tomato, almonds, cherries, and beans. Add the basil.

Per Serving: 204 calories, 9 g protein, 33 g carbohydrates, 9 g fat

MAIN DISHES
CILANTRO GRILLED SALMON

Makes 4 servings

4 wild salmon fillets (6 ounces each)
Sea salt
Freshly ground black pepper
2 tablespoons olive oil
1 lemon, juiced
1 cup cilantro, chopped

1. Preheat the grill to high. Place the salmon in a large piece of nonstick foil on the nonstick side and season with salt and pepper.
2. Mix together the oil, lemon juice, and cilantro. Drizzle the mixture over the salmon.
3. Close the foil and cook the salmon for 15 minutes, or until it flakes easily with a fork.

Per Serving: 307 calories, 34 g protein, 2 g carbohydrates, 18 g fat

LEMON HONEY MAHI MAHI

Makes 4 servings

3 tablespoons honey

2 tablespoons reduced-sodium soy sauce

1 lemon, juiced

¼ cup balsamic vinegar

1 clove garlic, minced

2 teaspoons olive oil

Sea salt

Freshly ground black pepper

4 mahi mahi fillets (6 ounces each)

1 tablespoon almond oil

1. Mix together the honey, soy sauce, lemon juice, balsamic vinegar, garlic, and olive oil in a shallow dish. Salt and pepper the fillets, then place them in a dish skin side down. Cover and refrigerate for 25 minutes.
2. Heat the almond oil on medium-high heat in a large skillet. Remove the fish from the dish, reserving the marinade. Cook the fish for 5 to 6 minutes on each side, turning once, or until it flakes easily with a fork. Remove from the skillet.
3. Add the reserved marinade to the skillet and heat on medium until it appears as a glaze. Drizzle the glaze over the fish and serve.

Per Serving: 375 calories, 32 g protein, 15 g carbohydrates, 20 g fat

WHOLE WHEAT LINGUINE WITH SHRIMP

Makes 4 servings

1 package (8 ounces) whole wheat linguine

1 teaspoon macadamia nut oil

6 cloves garlic, minced

1 cup reduced-sodium chicken broth

½ cup white wine

1 lemon, juiced

¼ teaspoon lemon peel

½ teaspoon freshly ground black pepper

Sea salt

1 pound fresh shrimp, peeled and deveined

2 teaspoons coconut oil

2 tablespoons fresh basil, chopped

1 cup fresh baby spinach, chopped

½ cup cherry tomatoes

1. Prepare the linguine according to package directions.
2. Heat the macadamia nut oil over medium heat in a large saucepan. Add the garlic and sauté for 1 to 2 minutes. Add the broth, wine, lemon juice, lemon peel, pepper, and salt. Simmer until reduced by half.
3. Add the shrimp, coconut oil, basil, and spinach to the saucepan. Cook for 2 to 4 minutes, or until the shrimp are heated through. Pour over the pasta and add the cherry tomatoes. Toss gently.

Per Serving: 420 calories, 40 g protein, 50 g carbohydrates, 8 g fat

CHICKEN CHILI WITH WHITE BEANS

Makes 6 servings

2 teaspoons almond oil

1 onion, chopped

3 cloves garlic, minced

4 cups reduced-sodium chicken broth

1 container (16 ounces) salsa verde

1 can (16 ounces) diced tomatoes, with juice

1 can (7 ounces) diced green chiles

½ teaspoon dried oregano

½ teaspoon chili powder

½ teaspoon ground cumin

1 pound cooked free-range chicken, diced

2 cans (15 ounces each) white beans

¾ cup frozen corn

Sea salt

Freshly ground black pepper

1. Heat the oil in a large stockpot. Sauté the onion and garlic until soft. Add the broth, salsa verde, tomatoes and juice, chiles, and spices. Bring to a boil, then reduce the heat and simmer for 10 minutes.
2. Add the chicken, beans, and corn. Simmer for 5 minutes. Add sea salt and pepper.

Per Serving: 331 calories, 34 g protein, 32 g carbohydrates, 6 g fat

FISH TACOS

Makes 5 servings (2 tacos per serving)

1 teaspoon almond oil

1 leek, chopped

3 cloves garlic, chopped

Sea salt

Freshly ground black pepper

¾ cup reduced-sodium chicken broth

2 large tomatoes, diced

2 teaspoons ground cumin

1½ pounds halibut fillets

1 fresh lime, juiced

10 corn tortillas

1. Heat the oil in a large skillet. Sauté the leek and garlic until soft. Add salt and pepper to taste.
2. Add the broth, tomatoes, and cumin to the skillet. Bring to a boil, and reduce heat to low. Add the halibut to the skillet and sprinkle with lime juice. Cover and cook the halibut for 15 to 20 minutes. Serve inside warm corn tortillas.

Variation: For a great sauce, mix some of the leftover fluid with light sour cream or a nondairy equivalent and drizzle over tacos.

Per Serving: 401 calories, 42 g protein, 41 g carbohydrates, 8 g fat

BLACK BEAN BURGERS

Makes 6 servings

2 cans (15 ounces each) black beans, drained and rinsed

1 ripe banana, mashed

1 onion, chopped

1 cup bread crumbs

1 scoop protein powder (hemp, pea, or rice)

2 cloves garlic, minced

2 tablespoons fresh basil

1 teaspoon dried oregano

1 teaspoon ground cumin

Sea salt

Freshly ground black pepper

6 whole wheat hamburger buns

1. Mash the black beans and banana in a medium bowl. Add the onion, bread crumbs, protein powder, garlic, basil, oregano, cumin, salt, and pepper, and mix well.
2. Form six patties and refrigerate for at least 30 minutes.
3. Heat a nonstick skillet to medium heat and spray with cooking spray. Carefully place the patties in the skillet and cook for about 4 minutes on each side, or until heated through.

Per Serving: 228 calories, 13 g protein, 40 g carbohydrates, 2 g fat

SIDES
BLACK BEANS WITH QUINOA

Makes 6 servings

1 teaspoon macadamia nut oil

1 onion, chopped

2 cloves garlic, minced

¾ cup quinoa, uncooked and rinsed

2 cups vegetable broth or reduced-sodium chicken broth

1 teaspoon ground cumin

Sea salt

Freshly ground black pepper

1 cup frozen corn

2 cans (15 ounces each) black beans, drained and rinsed

⅓ cup cilantro, chopped

1. Heat the oil in a medium saucepan. Sauté the onion and garlic until soft.
2. Add the quinoa, broth, cumin, salt, and pepper. Bring to a boil and then reduce the heat, cover, and simmer for about 15 minutes.
3. Add the frozen corn and simmer for another 3 to 5 minutes. Add the black beans and cilantro.

Per Serving: 236 calories, 11 g protein, 42 g carbohydrates, 3 g fat

BABY BOK CHOY WITH CASHEWS

1 tablespoon almond oil

2 cloves garlic, chopped

1 pound baby bok choy, rinsed with bases trimmed

½ teaspoon sesame oil

Sea salt

½ cup cashews

1. Heat the almond oil on medium heat in a large sauté pan. Add the garlic and bok choy. Sprinkle on the sesame oil and salt. Cover. Allow the bok choy to cook down for 3 to 4 minutes.
2. Add the cashews.

Per Serving: 151 calories, 4 g protein, 9 g carbohydrates, 12 g fat

EASY STEAMED SPINACH

Makes 4 servings

1 pound fresh baby spinach
Sea salt

1. Put the spinach in a stockpot and sprinkle with water. Place over medium heat.

2. Allow the spinach to cook down for 4 to 6 minutes and then sprinkle with sea salt.

Per Serving: 26 calories, 3 g protein, 4 g carbohydrates, 0 g fat

QUICK QUINOA

Makes 4 servings

1 teaspoon macadamia nut oil

4 cloves garlic, chopped

1 yellow onion, chopped

1 cup quinoa, uncooked and rinsed

2 cups vegetable broth or reduced-sodium chicken broth

3 tablespoons fresh basil

¼ teaspoon sea salt

½ lemon, juiced

1. Heat the oil in a saucepan. Sauté the garlic and onion until soft. Add the quinoa and broth. Bring to a boil. Reduce heat, cover, and simmer for 15 minutes.
2. Lightly toss together the quinoa, basil, and salt in a bowl. Sprinkle the lemon juice on the quinoa and serve.

Variations: Add ¼ cup slivered almonds. Refrigerate and add ¼ cup dried cranberries.

Per Serving: 197 calories, 7 g protein, 35 g carbohydrates, 4 g fat

EASY ASPARAGUS

Makes 4 servings

1 tablespoon almond oil
2 cloves garlic
4 tablespoons balsamic vinegar
Sea salt
1 pound asparagus

1. Preheat the oven to 425°F.
2. Mix the oil, garlic, balsamic vinegar, and sea salt in a small bowl. Transfer to a large sealable plastic bag. Put the asparagus in the plastic bag to coat.
3. Line a baking dish with foil and place the asparagus in a single layer.
4. Bake 6 to 8 minutes, or until done.

Per Serving: 70 calories, 3 g protein, 7 g carbohydrates, 4 g fat

SWEET POTATO FRIES

3 large sweet potatoes, peeled and sliced into ¼"-thick slices

2 tablespoons macadamia nut oil

½ teaspoon sea salt

Freshly ground black pepper

Pinch of ground red pepper

1. Preheat the oven to 425°F.
2. Sprinkle the potatoes with the oil and then toss them with the salt, black pepper, and ground red pepper.
3. Spread the potatoes in a single layer and bake for 10 minutes on each side, or until golden brown and soft on the inside.

Per Serving: 90 calories, 2 g protein, 14 g carbohydrates, 3 g fat

GUACAMOLE

Makes 8 servings

3 high-quality avocados (Hass)

1 lemon, juiced

1 tomato, diced

3 cloves garlic, chopped

1 teaspoon ground cumin

½ teaspoon sea salt

2 tablespoons cilantro, chopped

1. Cut the avocados into halves. After removing the seeds, scoop out the pulp and place it into a small bowl. Use a fork to mash the avocado.
2. Gently stir in the lemon juice, tomato, garlic, cumin, salt, and cilantro. Cover and refrigerate 1 hour prior to serving.

Per Serving: 116 calories, 2 g protein, 7 g carbohydrates, 10 g fat

BALSAMIC VINAIGRETTE

¾ cup balsamic vinegar

2 tablespoons high-quality extra-virgin olive oil

Combine the vinegar and oil. Mix well.

Per Serving: 45 calories, 0 g protein, 3 g carbohydrates, 3 g fat

DESSERTS
BERRY CRUMBLE

Makes 8 servings

2 cups blueberries

3 cups fresh strawberries, quartered

½ cup whole wheat flour

½ cup rolled oats

1 teaspoon cinnamon

2 tablespoons organic sugar

2 tablespoons agave nectar

1 tablespoon coconut oil

1. Preheat the oven to 375°F. Lightly coat a 13" x 9" baking dish with cooking spray.
2. Mix the blueberries and strawberries, and put them in the baking dish.
3. Mix together the flour, oats, and cinnamon in a medium bowl. Then add the sugar, agave nectar, and coconut oil until crumbly. Sprinkle the crumble topping over the fruit.
4. Bake for 25 minutes. Spoon into dishes and serve warm.

Per Serving: 130 calories, 3 g protein, 26 g carbohydrates, 2 g fat

AÇAÍ QUINOA DESSERT

Makes 4 servings

¾ cup quinoa, uncooked and rinsed

10.5 ounces Sambazon Açaí Juice

¼ cup dried cherries or cranberries

1. Add the quinoa, juice, and cherries or cranberries to a saucepan and cook over medium heat for 15 to 20 minutes, or until the liquid has been absorbed and the quinoa is cooked.
2. Chill for at least 1 hour before serving.

Per Serving: 190 calories, 4 g protein, 38 g carbohydrates, 3 g fat

PART 2 THE ULTIMATE FITNESS PROGRAM

CHAPTER 8

EATING FOR PERFORMANCE

"ALWAYS BEAR IN MIND THAT YOUR OWN RESOLUTION TO SUCCEED IS MORE IMPORTANT THAN ANY OTHER ONE THING."

—Abraham Lincoln

Exercise and nutrition are equally important when you are trying to build muscle and lose fat. The All-Pro Diet from Part 1 will help you maximize your workouts, as the food is healthy and will provide clean fuel to burn while you exercise. But the key to success is the precise timing of that fueling. Before we get to the workout program in this section, I'd like to give you some tips on how to time your eating (and drinking!) for top performance.

PREPARING FOR THE WORKOUT

If you exercise early in the morning, Mitzi suggests having a light snack such as a piece of fruit or an energy bar like a CLIF Nectar, LÄRABAR, Gnu, Zing, PURE Bar, or YouBar.

If you exercise later in the day, plan to have a small meal about 2 hours before you begin. I recommend a good source of whole grain carbohydrates, low in fat, moderate in protein and fiber. About 1 to 2 hours before exercise, you could have a snack such as an energy bar or a small (8- to 12-ounce) smoothie. Aim to always begin an exercise session in a fully hydrated state, so drink plenty of fluids.

If you're trying to lose weight, it's important to remember that you want to end each day with a calorie deficit—that is, simply burning up more calories than you take in. If your plan is to go to the gym and burn about 600 calories, it doesn't make sense to take in a lot of unnecessary calories preworkout or postworkout, as that can sabotage your weight-loss efforts.

Some people find that if they eat before exercising, they feel nauseated during the workout. Yet you need to be properly fueled and hydrated to effectively complete a workout. So try to find foods or drink that won't make you uncomfortable. You may have to experiment with some different options to see what works best for you.

DRINK UP!

If you watch football regularly, you have likely seen players leave the game and enter the locker room to get a bag of fluids through an IV.

WHAT TO EAT AND DRINK BEFORE TRAINING OR GAMES

Good Choices
Smoothie (not a huge one; about 8 to 12 ounces)

Fruit

Clean energy bar like PURE Bar, CLIF Nectar, LÄRABAR, Zing

Sports drink

One-half of a peanut butter and jelly sandwich

Bowl of cereal with lowfat milk

Poor Choices
Soda

Chips

Bacon

Whole milk

Cheeseburger

French fries

Milkshake

Dehydration definitely happens. Even during Super Bowls there have been instances where players started cramping and required treatment. Talk about negatively impacting performance! You can't perform if you aren't even on the football field.

Calculating Your Basic Water Needs

You must be hydrated to perform at your best. You have fluid in almost every space between your cells, and those cells function most efficiently when you've had enough fluids. Water eases proper digestion and it also cools your body. Remember, if you're exercising, your engine will run at a higher temperature than usual (muscles produce more heat during exercise), and water is the solution to keeping things cool and running smoothly.

As I've mentioned, a good way to determine your water requirements is to take your body weight in pounds and divide by 2. That's an estimate of the number of ounces of water you need each day. But if you're active, you need to increase your overall intake. If you don't want to have to calculate your fluid intake, just make sure you are drinking very regularly. Don't wait until you are thirsty because that means you are already dehydrated.

NATA FLUID REPLACEMENT GUIDELINES

The National Athletic Trainers' Association makes the following fluid recommendations:

- Drink 17 to 20 ounces 2 to 3 hours before practice or a game.

- Drink 7 to 10 ounces about 10 to 20 minutes before practice or a game.

- Drink 7 to 10 ounces every 10 to 20 minutes during exercise.

- After practice or a game, drink enough to replace any weight loss from exercise. You need about 20 ounces for every pound of weight lost.

Fueling Up During Your Workout

Athletic trainers are constantly preaching to their athletes that they need to consume plenty of sports drinks during training and competition. Often their athletes just aren't drinking enough to replace the fluids they've lost from sweating. Eventually, if they lose too much sodium through their sweat, they develop something called hyponatremia. This is when the level of sodium in the blood gets too low.

Mitzi suggests to players that, during games, they only consume sports drinks. Sports drinks provide calories to help maintain blood sugar levels, as well as sodium. They also taste better to most athletes, which encourages them to drink more. Trainers also use GatorLytes—packets of sodium they can add to increase the sodium concentration. (They are not commercially available, but if you are an Ironman triathlete, you definitely know what I'm talking about.) One commercially available alternative is a salt tablet, which can help some athletes who have high sweat rates and those who are involved in endurance sports.

While potassium is important, too, potassium loss is not a common problem, and you really don't need to worry about that if you are just going to the gym for an hour or so. Mitzi has told me that, unfortunately, there are still some coaches of young soccer, baseball, and softball teams who don't allow their athletes to drink sports drinks during

MITZI ADVISES . . .

Mitzi suggests that everyone trying to lose weight and doing short workouts of 1 hour or less carry a water bottle at the gym. This gives you a better estimation of your fluid requirements than drinking from a water fountain. By using a water bottle, you can accurately estimate your daily water intake. (Most water bottles are approximately 16 ounces.) Many people overestimate the amount of water they consume at a fountain, so the water bottle gives you a far more accurate measure, which is especially useful for young athletes. Also, aim for your urine to look more like lemonade than apple juice.

practice or competition. This is not a good idea, and definitely not what the science tells us.

Additionally, research has indicated that consuming a sports drink during weight training sessions may lower cortisol levels. Cortisol levels are especially important for strength athletes. As your workout becomes more difficult, more cortisol is released, and it can have a negative catabolic effect because it causes muscle protein breakdown. For the competitive athlete, I recommend sipping 14 to 20 ounces of Accelerade or Gatorade during a strength-training session to help decrease your cortisol levels, minimize muscle damage, and reduce immune system suppression.

There are some other reasons, as well, why athletes want to fuel up during exercise. It helps you maintain adequate blood glucose levels, replenish fluids and electrolytes, preserve muscle glycogen, and minimize muscle damage. Of course, any drinks or snacks you have during training or games should be part of the All-Pro Diet. Recharge your batteries with some fruit or with a clean energy bar. Always steer clear of sodas or other drinks containing high-fructose corn syrup and energy bars with ingredient lists a mile long.

WARNING SIGNS

I recommend that you weigh yourself without clothes before and after exercise so you can get an idea of how much fluid you are losing. Then develop your own individualized rehydration plan. Here are five warning signs of dehydration:

- Bright color and strong odor in your urine
- Fatigue
- Flushed skin
- Light-headedness
- Loss of appetite

If you are trying to lose weight or maintain your current weight, it is probably unnecessary for you to eat during exercise that lasts less than 60 minutes.

MY IDEAL RECOVERY NUTRITION PLAN

Anyone who wants to build muscle needs to pay attention to their *recovery* nutrition plan. It's the most important part of your diet if you're reaching toward weight loss and muscle-building goals.

Immediately following exercise, blood flow to the muscles will tend to peak. In fact, the first 15 to 30 minutes following exercise is the critical time to refuel because your muscles soak up glucose like a sponge. Even if you just wait a few hours before you fuel up again, the delay can impair recovery. By consuming the proper nutrients following exercise, your body will be better prepared to train the following day. You will also have less muscle soreness.

A lot of research has been conducted to find the optimal combination of nutrients that athletes need for recovery. Most research suggests the ideal ratio of carbohydrates to protein is somewhere between 2:1 and 4:1. In other words, shoot for drinking at least 50 grams of carbohydrates and about 15 grams of protein within 15 to 30 minutes following exercise.

YOUR RECOVERY NEEDS

I make it super simple for myself and just have Accelerade. If you are a numbers person and want specifics, here's how you can calculate your approximate carbohydrate and protein recovery needs for the first 30 minutes following exercise:

Carbohydrates

You'll need 0.5 gram of carbohydrates for every pound of body weight. For me that translates into 125 grams of carbohydrates. If you weigh in at 150 pounds, your needs are 0.5 x 150 pounds = 75 grams of carbohydrates. Keep in mind, if you are trying to lose weight, it's important to find the right balance of calories. You need enough to help your muscles recover while not taking in so many that you sabotage any weight loss efforts. In other words, it's probably not a good idea to crush 800 calories after a workout if your goal is weight loss.

Protein
Figure 0.23 gram of protein per pound of body weight. For a 150-pound person, that would be 0.23 x 150, or 34.5 grams of protein.

FOR RECOVERY—LIQUIDS OR SOLIDS?

While whole foods should be the foundation of your regular diet, during the recovery phase there are some definite benefits to choosing liquids over whole foods. First of all, liquids are digested more easily and absorbed more quickly. It can take a meal 2 to 4 hours to be digested, while a liquid supplement can be absorbed in 20 to 60 minutes! Since you want to consume your calories immediately after exercise, liquid nutrition is typically better tolerated and often more quick and convenient than whole foods.

After training or after a game, I always drink Accelerade. It uses a whey protein, but I like the perfect combination of carbohydrates and protein in the drink with its 4:1 ratio. A 12-ounce portion contains 120 calories, 21 grams of carbohydrates, and 5 grams of protein. I typically use three scoops. You can also make yourself a smoothie (see the recipes in Chapter 7).

Research has also shown some interesting anti-inflammatory benefits with tart cherries. The recovery juice below combines those benefits with the carbs and protein needed for recovery.

RECOVERY DRINK OPTIONS

Accelerade

Any of the All-Pro Smoothies from Chapter 7, but cut the recipes in half for recovery

Tony's Morning Power Smoothie

Mitzi's Berrylicious Smoothie

Oatmeal Berry Bliss Smoothie

Banana Berry Smoothie

Peach Mango Smoothie

Chocolate Banana Smoothie

12 ounces fat-free or 1% organic chocolate milk

Natural Recovery by CherryPharm

Pure Sport

Keep with the All-Pro Diet when you're selecting recovery foods. Stay away from the soda machine if you're thirsty, and don't eat chips, fast food, or high-fat foods. Just because you've been working out doesn't mean there's any reason to grab these health-damaging, performance-impairing foods.

MITZI ADVISES . . .

There are five good reasons to pay attention to recovery. Eating and drinking the right foods after you exercise . . .

1. Minimizes fatigue associated with repeated days of heavy training
2. Reduces muscle soreness
3. Prepares your muscles for maximum growth (an anabolic state)
4. Rehydrates after a tough workout
5. Replenishes muscle glycogen stores

UNLEASH THE POWER OF INSULIN NATURALLY

Most people neglect one of the most natural ways to take advantage of the increased activity of the anabolic hormones after exercise. Immediately after exercise, your anabolic hormones such as insulin, insulin-like growth factor-1 (IGF-1), testosterone, and growth hormone are elevated. Consuming a drink combining both carbohydrates and protein has been shown to produce a benefit by further increasing the levels of anabolic hormones and insulin. This is an ideal opportunity to replenish your glycogen and optimize muscle growth.

MITZI'S TOP 7 TIPS TO BUILD MUSCLE NATURALLY

One of the most common questions that I get, other than "How can I lose body fat?," is "How can I gain weight/build muscle?" This is especially common when high school boys are wanting to make the jump to collegiate athletics. I obviously promote gaining weight in a legal and natural way. The key to gaining weight for both the average Joe and for professional athletes is combining a good strength-training program like Tony's All-Pro Workout with a muscle-building nutrition plan. This nutrition plan means taking in *extra* calories. It takes approximately 2,500 additional calories to build 1 pound of muscle, so the overall goal is to increase your total calorie intake on a daily basis. The All-Pro Diet recommends these additional calories come from nutrient-rich sources of food: It's definitely not a free pass to eat junk food. Here are some of my tips on building muscle the natural way:

1. Never skip meals. Eat several times throughout the day.
2. Aim to eat at least an additional 400 to 500 calories each day. (Some athletes need to increase by 800 to 1,000 calories per day.)
3. Sometimes you will need to eat even when you are not hungry.
4. Always have a recovery drink with protein and carbohydrates after your workouts.
5. Increase your protein intake to about 0.8 or 0.9 gram per pound of body weight and stick with the All-Pro Diet protein sources.
6. Increase your intake of whole grains.
7. Increase your intake of healthy fats from foods like walnuts, avocados, and salmon.

SPECIFIC NUTRITIONAL STRATEGIES TO INCREASE CALORIE INTAKE

1. Add any All-Pro Diet smoothie as an extra snack during the day.
2. Add 1 or 2 peanut butter and honey or peanut butter and jelly sandwiches to your diet daily (reminder: whole wheat bread, natural peanut butter).
3. Mix together your favorite dried fruit with nuts (example: dried cherries or cranberries with raw almonds).
4. Add an extra All-Pro Diet–approved energy bar to your daily intake.

CHAPTER 9

PRIMED FOR PEAK PERFORMANCE

"TONY GONZALEZ IS ONE OF THE HARDEST WORKING FOOTBALL PLAYERS I'VE EVER MET."

—Herm Edwards, Former Coach of the Kansas City Chiefs

Now that you are on board with the All-Pro Diet, it's time to get serious about training for a better physique and building the power and strength that translates to playing better football or any sport. Based on all my trial-and-error lifting programs and from working with different strength coaches, I've come back with the ultimate workout. In 6 to 8 weeks of consistent training, this is a program that will whip you into top shape.

For any football player—offense or defense—this workout is the greatest. But it's not just for football players, either. Go ahead and use this program, and no matter what your sport, I'll bet you get results like never before. Follow this program with discipline, do the hard work, and I guarantee you'll be up to any physical challenge that you have to face on the field, on the court, or in the gym. This is how you can really excel.

I do my thing in the weight room during the season, then train on my own at my home in Southern California during the off-season. In that respect, I'm kind of an exception from most of the guys in the NFL. For instance, I'd say about 90 percent of the guys on my team live here on a year-round basis, so they use the team's strength-training facility. Some guys are contractually paid to do the off-season workouts at the team facility, while for other players it's more like, "You'd better stay here and do the program if you want to make the team."

I don't do the same workout as the guys who train at the team facility during the winter and spring. My version is a throwback to what the team used to do in the off-season when Jeff Hurd (now the strength and conditioning coach for the San Diego Chargers) was our strength coach when I was in Kansas City.

> ### "OUR GREATEST WEAKNESS LIES IN GIVING UP. THE MOST CERTAIN WAY TO SUCCEED IS ALWAYS TO TRY JUST ONE MORE TIME."
>
> —Thomas Edison

My off-season strength-training program begins when the season ends. From then until 50 days before training camp begins, I'll train two to three times per week, or four times if I'm trying to take it to a higher level of intensity. I do my training at home most of the time. I might lift weights when I play pickup basketball at a 24 Hour Fitness gym. It's a matter of what's most convenient and effective.

I'll hit the program harder and train *at least* 4 days a week once I'm 50 days out from camp. At that stage, I start doing a little bit more and I start pushing myself to lift heavier, get stronger.

Check out the photos on pages 179–196, and you can see that intensity is the name of the game for me when I'm pumping iron. The plan is to train Monday and Tuesday, take Wednesday off, and come back Thursday and Friday. I'll also play basketball on one of those days to focus on my cardiovascular conditioning regimen.

TRAINING TO BE ALL-PRO

My objective is to select exercises that carry over to the football field, but you'll also find them very effective in building a strong, athletic physique. Many of my strength-training movements are identical to the athletic movements I do as a pro football player; the only difference is that in the gym I have weights, instead of a football, in my hand. (Oh, another difference: I'm not getting pounded into the ground!)

Any lift or exercise has to be sport-specific. If you are a baseball player, you can use the medicine ball to simulate the swing: The physical action is bringing hips and hands to the ball. As a football player, what I want to do with the med ball is throw it against a wall using a side-to-side, hip-and-hands-to-the-ball type of motion. There are more than 100 different ways to throw a med ball that will help give you a great workout. It's terrific prep for any sport. When I do a power clean, the

---

Enjoy Wii—*and* Lose Weight!

I realize the program described in this chapter might not be for everyone. Just remember, nearly any kind of exercise will help you build muscle and lose weight if you're on the All-Pro Diet. For instance, anyone who has fun playing Nintendo Wii games will be glad to discover there's real calorie burn to help you lose weight. Here is what the benefits look like:

WII SPORT	CALORIES BURNED
Boxing	7.2 cal/min
Tennis	5.5 cal/min
Baseball	4.3 cal/min
Bowling	3.1 cal/min
Golf	2.3 cal/min

ultimate total-body blaster, the physical demands are akin to football; it's compatible with coming off the line of scrimmage and putting my hips into the movement.

VISUALIZING

Every time I'm lifting, I conjure a mental image of doing the exact same movement on the football field. Even if it's not the same exact movement, I use the mind-muscle connection to transfer what I'm doing in the gym to what I need to do on the football field. When I'm doing a squat, for instance, I visualize an Oakland Raider defensive back trying to tackle me while I'm trying to get up and out of the tackle. In my mind, I can also picture using the squat to help me block.

The mind-muscle connection is a matter of getting a mental image of doing something physical. When that image becomes crystal clear in your mind, your body will complete the picture with the correct movement. This is incredibly important. And it really works. I tell this to young players all the time. At first I'm not sure whether or not they believe me. So my advice is, try it! *Play the game before the game.* Go over the whole thing in your mind. Think about what you're going to do out there, how you're going to react if someone makes a certain move. See yourself going through all the plays. Take your time. Do the mental work.

Once you try it, there's no turning back. You realize that this carries over into everything you do. Not just sports. If you see something before it happens, then you've already been there in your mind, and you're totally ready.

> **"KNOWING IS NOT ENOUGH; WE MUST APPLY.**
> **WILLING IS NOT ENOUGH; WE MUST DO."**
>
> —Johann Wolfgang von Goethe, German Playwright

CHANGE IS ESSENTIAL TO SUCCESS

The exercises in my workout change every year. In fact, the program changes all the time. I vary my workouts frequently to avoid hitting a training plateau where I stop seeing results. I'll rotate exercises in and out of the routine to keep things fresh.

Sometimes I drop an exercise then find I have to bring it back again. I stopped doing squats for 2 or 3 years, and I started doing leg presses instead. The decision to dump squats was a mistake, because leg presses are not conducive to football. Leg presses are too stable; you are locked into a fixed position in the machine and no balance is brought into play.

I didn't know that at first. But when I gave up squats and just did leg presses, after a while I kind of noticed I was getting my butt kicked.

There's nothing like getting your butt kicked to help you figure out you've got to start doing something different. I figured it out. Those leg presses weren't giving me what I needed. My game suffered. Maybe it took me a while to catch on, but when I did, I was quick to give up something that wasn't working. I started doing squats again. My game started coming back. Results—right where I wanted them.

And that's the way you've got to work. If you're not getting the results, you'd better tweak your workout. It's the only way you're going to

---

A WORD TO THE WISE

I definitely recommend that you don't just jump right into all these exercises, especially if they are completely new to you. Make sure you get the help of a qualified strength and conditioning coach or personal trainer. Some good certifications to look for are CSCS, NSCA, and ACSM. You definitely want someone who knows what they are talking about and who can observe to make sure you have proper form. Some of these exercises might take a little time to build up to. Remember, I've been training my body for many years, and with all these exercises, I had to build up to where I am today. So don't overdo it too quickly.

improve. Oh, and by the way, I never went back to doing leg presses. With squats, it's just you and that bar on your back. You have to be able to control that bar. Your core (abdominal muscles and lower back) has to be fired up. With leg presses, you are sitting down on a slide and the weight is not going anywhere. During squats, when the weight is resting on your upper back, you have to carry and control it. That movement carries over to the football field way more than leg presses.

I'm here to tell you that free weights are better than machines for improving athletic performance. I've eliminated all machines from my workout routine, as it does not translate to the playing field. Pullups, which depend on using only your body weight for resistance, are superior to wide-grip pulldowns. I prefer pullups because they're more effective at increasing functional back strength. Machines are for shaping, not for improving athleticism.

TONY G.'S ULTIMATE ALL-PRO WORKOUT
THE PRE-WEIGHT TRAINING WARM-UP

My favorite warm-up movement is jumping rope. Jeff Hurd, my former strength coach, told me it was one of the best workouts you can do for cardio and overall physical conditioning. Boxers use this exercise to stay light on their feet. Jumping rope fires up your calf muscles (gastrocnemius and soleus), tones shoulders, and enhances full-body coordination to make you more graceful on the football field.

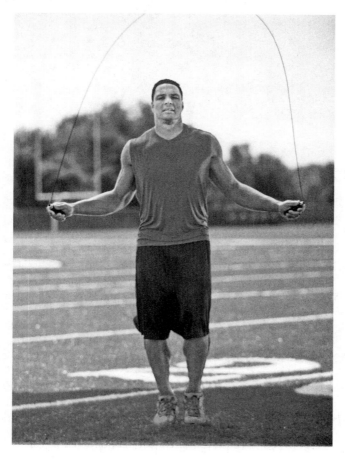

JUMP ROPE: 600 to 1,000 jumps total, 100 jumps per set, 30 seconds of rest between sets. This helps keep the feet quick.

CRUNCHES (250 reps in total): 1 set of 100 reps, straight crunches; 1 set of 100 reps, side crunches; 1 set of 25 reps, straight crunches; 1 set of 25 reps, side crunches.

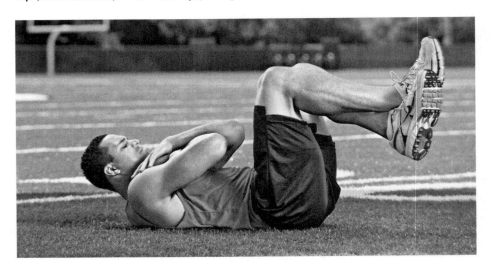

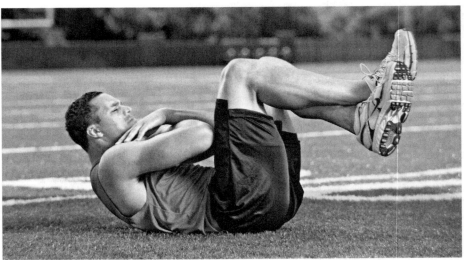

STRAIGHT CRUNCHES: Lie flat on your back with your chin tucked down on your sternum. Place your hands either behind your head or across your chest. The goal is to keep your chin down, because it helps keep your abs flexed the whole time. Raise your shoulder blades off the floor and keep your abs contracted. Roll up toward your knees; your feet are off the floor in an L-position. Slowly lower and repeat. Exhale on the contraction.

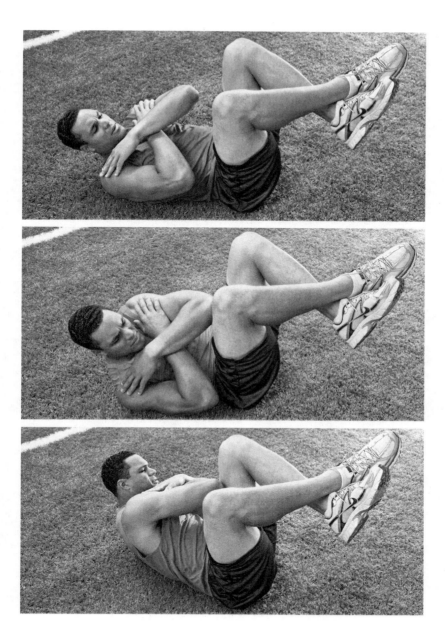

SIDE CRUNCHES: Lie on your back; rotate from elbow to opposite knee.

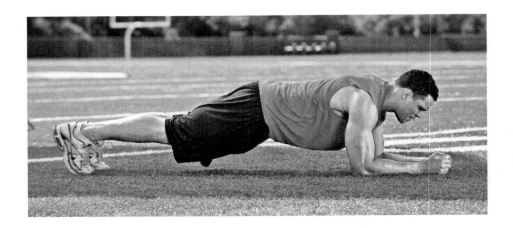

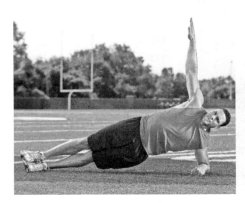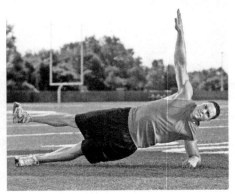

YUGO (aka bridges or planks): A yoga exercise that relies on your body weight for resistance. I'll do different poses without resting. It hits your core and lower back.

Get into a pushup position, but rest your weight on your forearms instead of your hands so that your body forms a plank. Contract your abdominals and hold for 1 minute. (You can start with 30 seconds and work your way up to 1 minute.)

Variation: Rotate to your left side—one arm stays down on the floor and the other arm comes up in the air—until your body is parallel to the floor. Your left forearm is flat on the floor and you try to get your body parallel to the ground, but it will be at an angle because only the one forearm and your feet touch the floor. Hold for 30 to 60 seconds.

Variation: Now rotate to your right side in the same position, without letting anything but the forearm and feet touch the ground. Now raise your top leg so your feet are shoulder-width apart. Hold for 30 to 60 seconds. Rest and repeat the cycle three times.

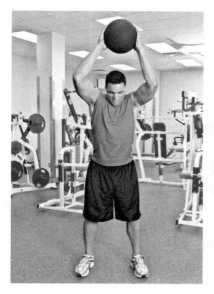
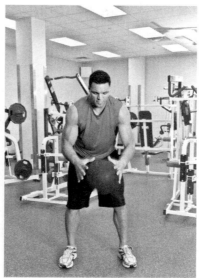
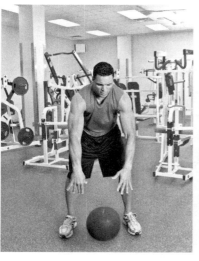
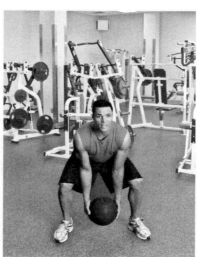

MEDICINE BALL THROW

Throw the med ball up in the air and catch it. Throw the ball over your head and from behind your head. Do as many reps as possible.

THE WEIGHT SESSION BEGINS

Set and rep ranges for all core movements (each training cycle lasts 2 weeks):

Cycle 1

Do three sets of 10 reps. Keep the weights fairly light.

Cycle 2

Do four sets of 8 reps.

Cycle 3

Do five sets of 5 reps.

Cycle 4

Go back up to 10 to 12 reps for three sets, but lower the weight a little bit. Keep the weight heavy enough to challenge yourself, but don't start out with the same weight you were using in Cycle 1 when you were doing lower reps. Once you can handle more reps with perfect form, you can build up to a heavier load again.

I'm going to show you how to do these tough exercises the right way to guarantee maximum gains while staying injury free. Check it out!

THE EXERCISES

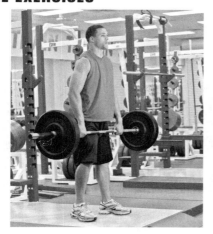
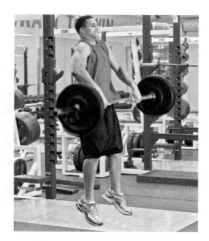
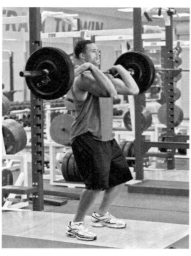
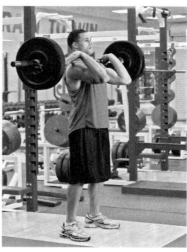

POWER CLEANS: Begin the lift in a basic athletic stance: Feet slightly past shoulder-width apart, chest and head up. Bend your knees as you would during squats. Explode with your legs; that raw power generated from the legs is what helps move the bar. Once you get the bar moving into a power-shrug position, pull with your arms (that's what we call the "clean" part of the movement) up to your collarbone and catch the weight while still in that solid athletic stance. The whole theory behind power cleans is triple extension: The movement starts in your feet, goes to your knees, and then projects through the hip. You get triple extension out of all those joints to move the weight. You can do power cleans with either barbells or dumbbells; personally, I like to alternate between these two free-weight options.

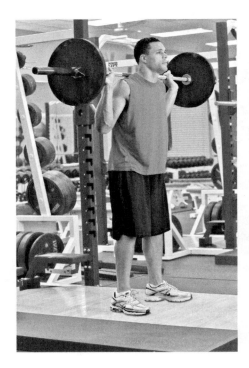
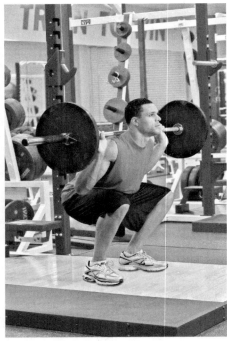

SQUATS are an overall strength-building movement for the quadriceps and hamstrings. Place your feet slightly wider than shoulder-width apart. Keep your shoulders back, chest up. Squat down to a parallel position (your thighs are parallel to the floor). Keep your knees right over your toes; don't let the knees point in or out. Make sure you don't round out your back. Return to the starting position and repeat.

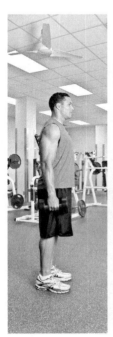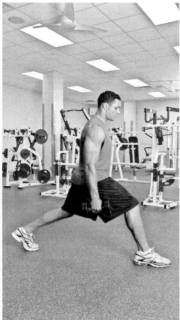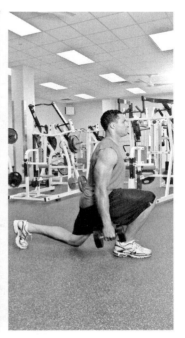

LUNGES work balance, quad and hamstring flexibility, and develop quickness with a stride-and-step movement. Start with your shin perpendicular to the floor and your quad parallel to the floor; your chest is up. Hold a set of light dumbbells for added resistance.

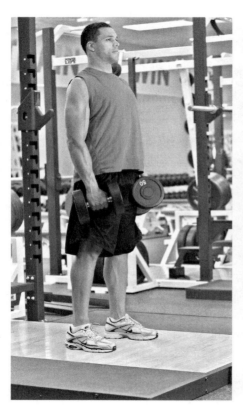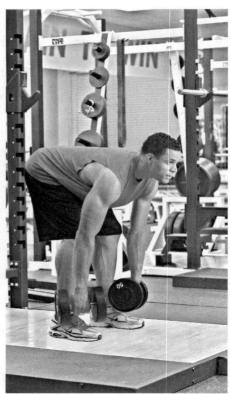

RDLs are isolation movements for the lower back, glutes, and hamstrings. Start with a low weight and make sure your posture is strong and stable. Start with the weight as if you were going to do a power clean, but instead lower it straight down about 3 inches above the floor. Slowly stand back up and repeat.

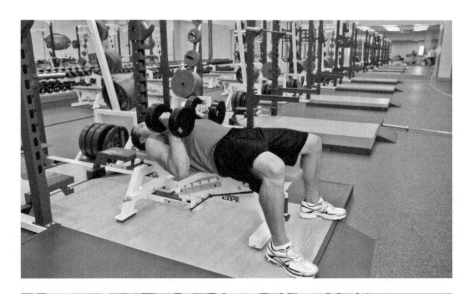

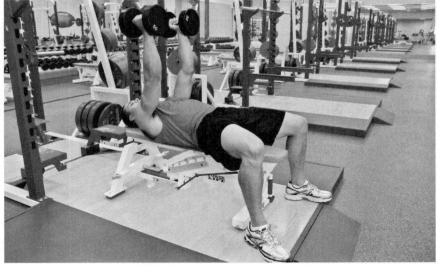

DUMBBELL BENCH PRESSES, in which you are forced to balance each dumbbell independently, transfer well to playing football because you get so one-handed on the football field. Lie down in a supine position on a flat bench. Lower the dumbbells until they touch the outside of your chest. Push the weights back up off your chest.

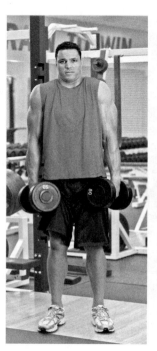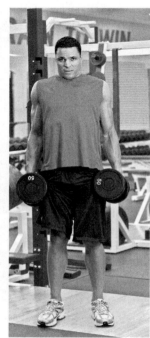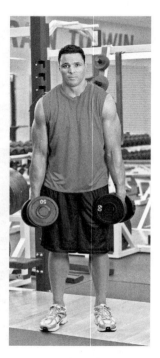

SHOULDER SHRUGS work your trapezius muscles. Hold a dumbbell in each hand and elevate your shoulders as high as possible toward your ears—keep your arms straight! Let your shoulders down slowly and then shrug them up for the next rep.

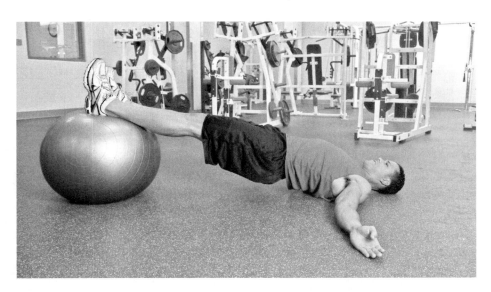

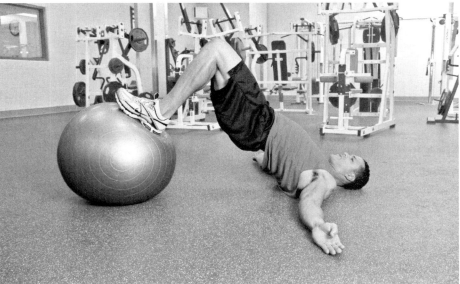

LEG CURLS on a stability ball target your hamstrings. Get in the plank position with your heels up on the stability ball—nothing touches the floor except for your shoulder blades and arms. Curl the ball toward your buttocks to work your hamstrings as you elevate your hips in the air. Starting position: Your heels are on the ball. Contracted position: When you finish, your feet are flat on top of the ball and the ball has been moved toward your butt. Straighten without letting your hips (or anything else but your arms and shoulders) touch the floor.

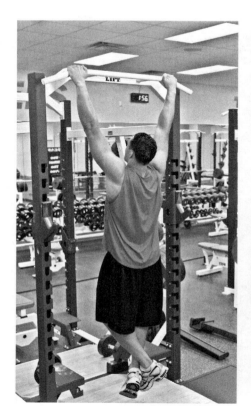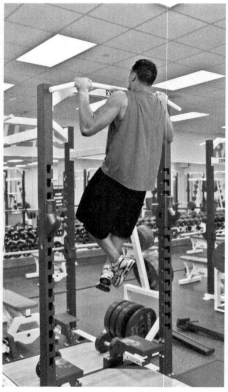

PULLUPS develop your upper body, especially shoulders (deltoids) and back (lats). Take a wide grip (just past shoulder-width), and when you are almost chinning the pullup bar, your forearms should be close to your body. When you pull up and get your chin over the bar, your forearms must be perpendicular (straight up) in relation to the floor.

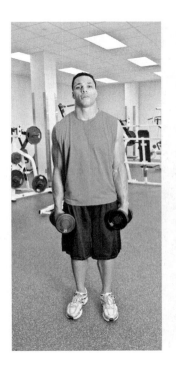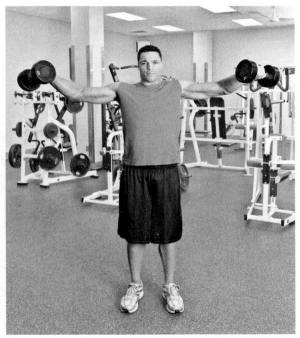

DUMBBELL LATERAL RAISES are great for toning side deltoids. Stand upright, balanced on your feet. Begin with the dumbbells in front of your waist. Now, raise the weights out to the sides, keeping a slight bend in the elbows, with your hands ending up on top of the dumbbell and at ear height. Bring the dumbbells back to the center of your body—in front of your waist.

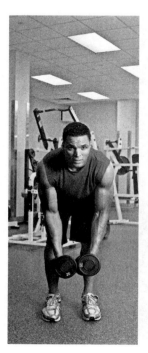
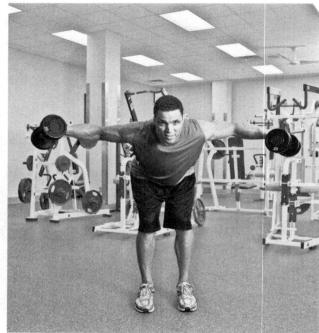

BENT-OVER LATERAL RAISES repeat the same exact movement as for lateral raises, but this time in an RDL posture: Your back is flat and parallel to the floor with your knees bent. Raise the dumbbells out to the side until they are parallel to the floor, with your hands on top of the dumbbells.

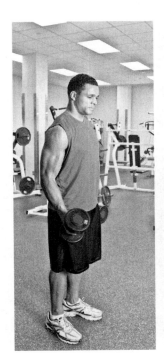 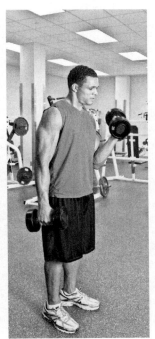 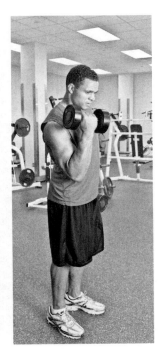

DUMBBELL CURLS strengthen the biceps, allowing you to perform a variety of movements and carry heavier loads. Start with dumbbells at your side—you can do this either seated or standing. Keeping your elbow close to your side, curl the dumbbell up toward your face.

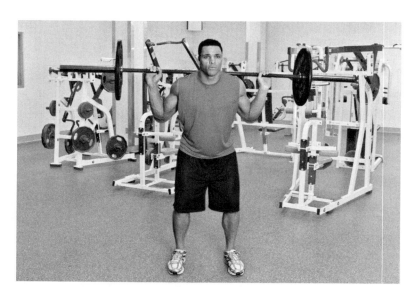

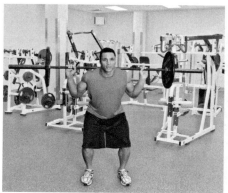

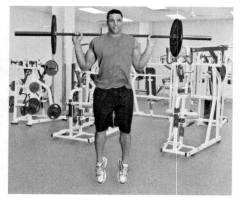

BOUNDERS are an exercise that I use to increase vertical leap. These are not part of the standard workout, but I want you to try them because they will improve your jumping and leaping ability. I put a straight bar with a light weight on my upper back and bound up and down for 12 to 15 reps. I visualize that I'm either jumping up to hit the boards for a rebound or leaping to catch a pass. I've got that weight pulling me down and it's a lot like being hit as I jump up in a crowd of defenders to catch the ball. When the weight is on my back, I'm not literally jumping off the floor; I'm simulating the movement of the jump, and it's a great way to work calves, glutes, hamstrings, and quads. Do five actual jumps without the bar as a warm-up to bounders. I guarantee that your vertical jump will improve.

ORGANIZING THE WORKOUT

I don't believe in splitting up my workout into upper and lower body sessions in alternate workouts. I hit my entire body in one workout.

CORE EMPHASIS

This workout is designed to work the core (abs, trunk, and lower back) in order to improve balance and strength. Mike Spirling, a good friend of mine who is now a trainer, taught me the importance of core training.

About 7 years ago, we were hanging out and having fun at my parents' house, throwing the football around. He told me to get up on one leg. And while I was trying to balance on one leg, he tapped me lightly on the side, and I fell over. That's when I knew my balance was poor, as my core was weak. Without balance, you will limit your full athletic potential.

THE SCHEDULE

I lift on Mondays (the day after a game) and I'll squat heavy. (Squatting before or after practice is very tough, so I like to do my squats on a day when we don't have practice.) I want to keep my leg strength, as that's my advantage on the football field. I want to do my bench press on Monday too. It will depend on what the coach gives me to do that day.

My off-season warm-up stays exactly the same during the season. I continue to jump rope and do the other core movements.

CHANGES IN THE WORKOUT WHEN THE SEASON BEGINS

The training sessions become shorter during the season. My goal is to maintain strength, not to unrealistically expect to build new strength while I'm playing football.

The objective is to maintain the strength that I have when training camp ends and the season begins. A player can get stronger during the season, but a lot will depend on injuries. If I hurt my shoulder, for instance, I won't be able to lift as heavy. If I hurt my knees, that will hurt my ability to squat with heavy weights.

"AS LONG AS YOU'RE GOING TO BE THINKING ANYWAY, THINK BIG."

—Donald Trump

QUALITY, NOT QUANTITY

In high school, lifting for football was all about how much weight a player could bench press and squat. There are guys on my team who can bench and squat way more weight than me, but when you put them on the football field, I will beat them every time.

It's important to have a strong bench press, but I don't need to bench 450 pounds. I don't have to bust my butt to bench that much; that's not going to help on the football field. Athleticism is far more important, for it will beat the stronger guy every time. I'm a firm believer that this rule carries over to every position, including offensive and defensive line.

Will Shields, a Pro Bowl guard, was not the strongest guy on our team in the weight room. That didn't make any difference because he was a great athlete.

You know what doesn't make sense? The practice of testing football players on the bench press to see how many reps they can crank out at 225 pounds. The amount you can bench press doesn't have anything to do with actual athletic ability or football skill.

I want good weight-room numbers. I'm concentrating on my athleticism. Typically, the guys with great weight-room numbers are missing out on their athleticism and are overlooking their core development, footwork, and vertical jump in order to get them. Those skills are all sports related. This is not the Summer Olympics, where the lifters are trying to break world records. I don't have any idea what my one-rep max would be on the bench press and I don't care.

DISCIPLINE MAKES THE DIFFERENCE

What I can't figure out is why NFL teams have their players work out hard during the off-season, then let the guys go out on their own 6 weeks before the season starts. I get the part about the guys wanting to take vacations and enjoy a break from the grind. What I don't get is how the team rationalizes the fact that the players are losing all these gains they made during the off-season workout program if they don't choose to work out during that off-time.

A player who lacks self-discipline will tend to do very little for those 6 weeks before training camp. I'll come to mini-camp during the off-season, and these guys are huge. I can tell they've been hitting the gym every day. And then as soon as the season rolls around, they are looking a lot smaller. By the time the season ends, they are even smaller.

It takes a lot of discipline to lift during the season, since you are also practicing for 1 hour and 45 minutes. Wednesday and Thursday practices are tough because you are in pads. After the game (on Monday, typically), you don't want to lift because you are sore and tired. And on Friday, you don't want to lift too much because you have another game coming up in 48 hours.

Many players, therefore, lift only twice per week. I lift three times per week, which is unusual. I lift Monday, Wednesday, and Friday and do the warm-up routine 5 days per week. I allow for 2 days off, Tuesday and Saturday, to mentally and physically recharge my batteries.

My former strength coach and mentor, Jeff Hurd, taught me the value of hard work in the weight room. I'm asking you to put out that same effort to make the strength gains you're looking for in your own gym workout. (I've let Jeff speak in his own words on page 221.)

The point is, there really is no way around hard work and discipline if you want to achieve the very top level of excellence and perform at your best all the time. I know I'm not the first person to say that. I've read a lot of biographies of great people (they're quoted in this book), and they all come back to the same point. If you want to be great, you have to have discipline. I guarantee it: *There is no other way!*

PART 3

THE ALL-PRO MINDSET FOR SUCCESS

CHAPTER 10

INTRODUCTION TO THE 8-POINT PLAN OF ATTACK

"ALL SUCCESSFUL COACHES AND PLAYERS HAVE AT LEAST ONE THING IN COMMON—A STRONG GAME PLAN."

—Lou Holtz, Author and Former NFL Head Coach

Now that you have followed through on the commitment to clean up your diet and train like a pro football player, it's time to fit in the last piece of the puzzle—the mental intensity you need to achieve all your goals in life.

I'm going to show you how to put your game face on and to learn from my experience in football. Each element of the mindset has helped me to play better and to be a more complete person. Here's the eight-point plan of attack that will help you reach the objectives you set for yourself.

I know this eight-point plan works for football players. But will it work for anyone? Absolutely! This isn't a specialized, narrow approach. It's the kind of approach that will help you reach all your objectives, no matter who you are or what you intend to achieve.

1. Read everything.

2. Surround yourself with good people.

3. Learn how to build personal relationships.

4. Set goals.

5. Work harder than the rest.

6. Live generously.

7. Have fun!

8. Take action.

I'll bet some of these points are already a big part of your life. Look at the fact that you've already read the book this far. Doesn't that say something about the way you want to change? You're really into it! Now, the challenge is to work on the areas where you need some additional concentration. I believe that all eight steps in this plan of attack need to be given a lot of effort. Here's why:

1. READ EVERYTHING.

It took me a while to discover the importance of reading up on things that were important to me. But when I did—what a difference!

Let me explain.

I didn't start for the Kansas City Chiefs my first season, but I had 33 catches and was used a lot in passing situations. It was my second season in Kansas City—my sophomore year—that really put my mental toughness to the test. It ranks right up there with my first football experience, in the Pop Warner league, that I mentioned in the introduction to this book. Even though I was starting and I was playing a lot, I dropped 17 passes and missed out on countless plays.

With about five games left in the season, I got a letter from my buddy Donnie Burger. This was totally out of the blue. He'd never sent me a letter before, so it was very surprising. The letter basically said, "Tony, I've been watching you play this year and there's something going on with you. I don't know what it is. What I do know is that you're not the Tony that you used to be. Just get back to being the old Tony—just be true to the real Tony."

He gave me a pamphlet that had a bunch of quotes from Vince Lombardi, one of the greatest coaches in NFL history. This was one of those defining moments in my life!

I read the pamphlet in about 20 minutes, and that inspired me to go to a bookstore (probably my first trip to search out a book in many years) to buy Vince Lombardi's book *When Pride Still Mattered*. I read the book in about a week, and I went through a complete transformation in my character. That book hit me with the complete mindset package. Lombardi wrote about confidence, hard work, and the attitude you need to maintain on the field. It was like he was talking directly to me about my own game. He preached the idea that there's no such thing as second place. He talked about the intangibles that go with being a good player.

Reading that book changed my whole season around. By then, though, it was too late for me to prove that I was different. The fans were calling me a bust. The newspapers were saying I was not as good as my hype. I was graded a D– in Jason Whitlock's analysis of the Chiefs by position. Whitlock, a football writer for the *Kansas City Star*, said the only reason I didn't get an F was because I had some good games at the end of the year. (That was when the mindset finally clicked for me.)

But I was embarrassed. I remember going out to dinner with some other guys from the Chiefs and overhearing the person behind us saying, "That guy Gonzalez sucks! He's horrible. I can't believe we ever drafted him." I'm a sensitive person, and I was very upset. I didn't think I was that bad. (That's why I feel bad for guys who get trashed in the media, because it makes it hard to go out. You feel like you're letting down your family.)

Still, I felt the difference in myself that had come about because of Lombardi's book. So, once the season was over, I started devouring self-help books. I read a book by Lou Holtz, the famous coach who now covers college football for ESPN, about success. Tony Robbins, Deepak Chopra, and Dr. Phil were all great inspirations to me. I would take notes and do a lot of thinking and reflecting after each book I read.

From self-help books, I moved on to the more spiritual books to teach me how to quiet my mind and improve my visualization—what I call vision. From these books I learned that visualization and being mentally focused are skills that develop over time. You have to be able to see yourself make the play in advance. You try to smell the ground around you. Put yourself in that third-and-long situation and figure out how you are going to make that play. How are you going to run that route? Once I learned how to do it, I would get really detailed in my vision. Now I'll do this all week long to prepare for the game. I'll work on visualization on the sidelines during practice. (Once I'm running a play, though, I'm in the moment and just focusing on being the best player I can be that day.)

And that turnaround all began with reading the right books!

2. SURROUND YOURSELF WITH GOOD PEOPLE.
Obviously, this is extremely important for pro athletes. But it's equally important for anyone in any line of work. And it's true in your personal life as well. I know why I've stayed out of trouble, and it's all because I hang out with good people. And I want to be around positive people. I automatically avoid negative people who are always complaining. I know how they always seem to bring you down.

"CHARACTER IS POWER."
—Booker T. Washington

3. LEARN HOW TO BUILD PERSONAL RELATIONSHIPS.

One of the highlights of my football career with the Kansas City Chiefs was playing for Coach Dick Vermeil, the most personable coach I've ever been around in my entire sporting life. Coach Vermeil treated every player on the team with complete respect.

Coach Vermeil always talked about the importance of relationships. "The relationship part of this business is the best part. Never forget to be generous with friendships," he told us.

Coach Vermeil and his wife, Carol, preached a humanistic approach to football. Whether you were the star player or the guy struggling to make the final roster cut, Coach would take the time and effort to talk to you and invite you over to his house for dinner. There, Coach and Carol Vermeil taught me a very important lesson about life—don't forget to care about the people you work with every day. Before that time, I'd pretty much stayed to myself and hadn't reached out to my teammates as friends. Now I came to understand that the mental side of football was actually having fun with it rather than treating it as a job.

Recapturing the fun in football was also an important step for me. The irony is that most athletes say they had the most fun when they played (for free!) in high school or college. In school sports, that's the mind-set—you play for fun, not money. No matter how long I play professionally, I hope I can always cherish the mindset that I had back then. I'm playing a kid's game and it should be fun—not a grind or simply a means to an end.

When you play for your teammates, for the fans, or for the love of the game, you will see better results. The same idea applies for everyone. Work goes so much faster when you actually love what you are doing and when you enjoy hanging out with the people you work with.

I have Coach Vermeil to thank for developing this kind of appreciation for the sport and helping me to realize that life is all about building meaningful relationships and caring about other people. He showed me what it means to value your friendships and treat all people with equal respect.

> **"I FOUND THAT THE MEN AND WOMEN WHO GOT TO THE TOP WERE THOSE WHO DID THE JOBS THEY HAD IN HAND, WITH EVERYTHING THEY HAD OF ENERGY AND ENTHUSIASM AND HARD WORK."**
>
> —Harry S. Truman

4. SET GOALS.

My All-Pro Mindset begins with setting goals for every aspect of my life. Each year, I start out by writing down all my goals on a piece of paper. Then I know what those goals are, and I lay out what I need to do to achieve each and every one of them.

A new football season demands a new set of goals. The plan is to make them as realistic as possible. In other words, I'm not shooting for 150 catches and 2,000 yards in receiving, because that's beyond what's possible. It's out of my reach. Similarly, a high school athlete who has never played football before and is trying out for the team for the first time should not expect to be the best player on the team. That's an unrealistic goal!

So what's realistic? It all depends on where you are at the moment and what you can accomplish in the time frame that you set for yourself. For my rookie season in the NFL, I remember setting a goal of 65 catches and 700 yards. What I actually achieved that year was 33 catches and about 300 yards. So—I didn't reach my goal. I didn't even come close. I knew I'd set my goals, but I also thought they were achievable. The fact that I didn't get there just meant I had to work harder.

Most of the time, I never hit *all* my goals. But I often come close. I set my goals high, but not off the charts.

One thing I like to do—and I recommend this for anyone being coached or mentored—is ask my coach, "What do you want from me this season? What do you expect?" Whatever answer he gives, I go a little bit beyond that. If he says, "75 catches, 1,000 yards, and 7 touchdowns," I'll come back and say to myself, "Okay, then I want 85 catches, 1,100 yards, and 10 touchdowns." And that becomes my personal goal for the season.

Over the years I've always increased my expectations for catches, touchdowns, and yardage. Through those years, though, I've been reluctant to share my goals with too many people. I don't want to brag about what I want to accomplish. That's not the point. I just want to make myself accountable for getting the job done—and have a plan of action to guide me along the way. The goals I set for myself include personal goals as well as objectives for my football season. A personal goal? It might be that I want to become a better husband this year. How am I going to do that? It takes work, patience, and caring. Without the goal of self-improvement, I wouldn't have a chance to be more considerate to my wife or become a better father.

In my opinion, every coach should have their players come up with a list of goals. There is amazing power in goal-setting. Writing down specific goals puts that information in your mind. It's up to you to keep working every single day to reach those goals. Hard work is essential if you plan to make improvements in your performance.

One thing I tell young athletes is to forget about looking forward to playing in the NFL some day. Stay in the present. Great athletes always find a way to remain totally focused in the moment. When I'm about to run a play, I'm not thinking about the next play or the last play. It's all about staying focused on *this one play*, in the *here and now*. The present is called the present for a reason, and that's because it's a gift.

Part of what got me to the NFL in the first place was this mindset. I learned to focus, to stay in the moment. I didn't worry about who was going to draft me or where I'd end up playing. I'm a firm believer that things have a way of taking care of themselves, providing you align yourself with good principles and good morals.

> ## "OBSTACLES ARE THINGS YOU SEE WHEN YOU
> ## TAKE YOUR EYES OFF YOUR GOAL."
>
> —E. Joseph Cossman, Author and Entrepreneur

5. WORK HARDER THAN THE REST.

It was Vince Lombardi who said, "The most competitive games draw the most competitive men."

Building self-confidence comes down to working harder and being hungrier than the next guy. I have seen many young players come and go in the NFL. All of them are talented. But many of those talented guys just mail it in. They stay for 3 years, and then they're gone. They don't work hard enough to stick around and improve.

> ## "THE ONLY PLACE YOU'LL FIND SUCCESS BEFORE WORK
> ## IS IN THE DICTIONARY."
>
> —May B. Smith

Working hard does have a direct correlation with being the best and building the confidence needed to get better. I study elite athletes like Michael Jordan, Lance Armstrong, Jerry Rice, and Tiger Woods. I analyze their approach to sports in order to understand what makes them great. Some people would say their approaches are a little crazy. I've heard stories about Tiger Woods from friends of mine who went to school with him at Stanford. In one story, they had played a night basketball game and were returning to campus at 1 a.m.—and there was Tiger hitting golf balls. He's always been like that. Tiger Woods will finish playing 18 holes and then play the entire course again later in the day. I wouldn't be surprised if he went back to the links the following morning to hit balls before his 7 a.m. tee time. Crazy stuff, but that's what helped to make him so great.

Michael Jordan's practice habits were unbelievable, too. "To see how far a commitment to excellence can take you, look no further than Michael Jordan," observes Lou Holtz, the great football coach at Notre Dame and the University of South Carolina. What Holtz admires, above all else, is Jordan's remarkable work ethic. "He is one individual I would want to have on any team I coached, whether basketball, football, golf, or whatever. Game in, game out, Jordan demands optimum effort from himself and his teammates. He can't stomach mediocrity. And while any-one with eyes can recognize Michael Jordan's talents, you should know that no one practices harder than this All-Star forward. He's always working to improve his game even though he's already the best player on the planet."

How many people have the discipline of a Michael Jordan or a Tiger Woods? Not many. But if you want to be great, I'm afraid you have to be willing to pay the price.

"WHEN A DIFFICULT TASK COMES YOUR WAY, ACCEPT THE CHALLENGE JOYFULLY. ONCE IT IS FINISHED, PLEAD FOR MORE. EVERY SACRIFICE YOU MAKE BUILDS CHARACTER. PEOPLE WITH AVERAGE SKILLS OFTEN OBTAIN GREATNESS BECAUSE THEY ARE WILLING TO PAY A PRICE FOR IT. YOU MIGHT NOT BE ABLE TO OUTTHINK, OUTMARKET, OR OUTSPEND YOUR COMPETITION, BUT YOU CAN OUTWORK THEM. YOU MAY BE ASKING WHY I THINK SACRIFICE IS VITAL TO ANY WINNING GAME PLAN. MY ANSWER IS SIMPLE: SO FEW PEOPLE ARE WILLING TO MAKE THEM. THOSE OF YOU WHO HABITUALLY DO THAT LITTLE BIT EXTRA WILL ENJOY A TREMENDOUS EDGE OVER THE COMPETITION."

—Lou Holtz

In my childhood I was a schoolyard legend in Huntington Beach, Cal-ifornia, and yet I hit a crisis of confidence when I tried out for Pop War-ner football in fifth grade. I was not getting a chance to play, so I decided to quit the team. During recess or gym class, I was the best football player in my school, but for some reason I couldn't make the grade in Pop Warner.

This is what I call my fifth-grade crisis. Back in elementary school, I had been unwilling to make that personal sacrifice to be good enough to make the team. I was not able to "do that little bit extra" to gain the edge. Several years later, I had a chance to try out for high school football and I was ready to go the extra step. When I showed up at football practice the first day, all the guys remembered me from Pop Warner, and they greeted me with skepticism: "Are you trying out again?" On my first day ever in pads, we were doing a full-pad drill in practice called Oklahoma, in which you had to pick a hole and hit the guy who was trying to plug the hole. Eric Escobido, the best and toughest player on the team and a good friend of mine, called me over from three rows back and told me to go up against him in the drill. We smashed into each other and it was a stalemate, a draw. I had built up my confidence and proved that I was willing to work hard to become a great football player.

> "A YOUNG PERSON, TO ACHIEVE, MUST FIRST GET OUT OF HIS MIND
> ANY NOTION EITHER OF THE EASE OR RAPIDITY OF SUCCESS.
> NOTHING EVER JUST HAPPENS IN THIS WORLD."
>
> —Edward Bok, Pulitzer Prize–Winning Author

It was all a matter of building self-confidence, getting myself right mentally, and believing I could do it. When you get older, having a well-developed work ethic becomes much more important. A CEO can't be afraid of hard work if he wants to keep his job. Any successful person has to develop self-confidence.

I like to use the football field as an example of the need to work hard in order to be the best. Everyone works hard in the NFL—that's a given. But what did you do before practice, and what did you do after practice? Those are the key questions. I always get to practice at least 15 minutes early to work on catching the ball, route running, and technique. When other players leave practice to take their showers, I stay on the field for an extra 15 minutes to work on catching the ball, route running, and technique—those same things I focused on before practice.

When I speak to kids, I tell them that no matter what you do in life, you will get out of it what you put into it. In sports, if you put in sorry effort, you will get sorry results. I guarantee it. But if you put in *great* effort on a consistent basis and are doing things the right way, there is no doubt in my mind that you will get *great* results!

> **"A DIFFICULT TIME CAN BE MORE READILY ENDURED IF WE RETAIN THE CONVICTION THAT OUR EXISTENCE HOLDS A PURPOSE—A CAUSE TO PURSUE, A PERSON TO LOVE, A GOAL TO ACHIEVE."**
>
> **—John Maxwell, Leadership Expert and Best-Selling Author**

6. LIVE GENEROUSLY.

What if you become great in your chosen field? How are you going to handle success?

I preach that the best way to handle success is by being humble and giving something back to your community. The goal in life is to give back to the people around you and to be genuine in caring for others. I'm not going to do charity work just because someone is telling me to do it. I donate my time to helping people because it means something to me.

To me, living generously simply means caring about other people. The best part is seeing the smiles after taking the time to show that you care. You can really touch a person with kindness, and that's especially true in my position as a professional athlete. Both adults and kids look up to professional athletes and treat us as role models. Giving back is one of the true pleasures of success. I started the Tony Gonzalez Foundation to help children and seniors with special needs. I visit hospitals and deliver Shadow Buddies to anyone—whether young or old—in need of companionship and friendship. (A Shadow Buddy is actually a doll that has the same ailment the kid is suffering from.) Working with the Shadow Buddies and the kids who need help allows me to show compassion and love for sick kids and lonely seniors.

My foundation is not about finding a cure for disease; instead, it is focused on making people comfortable and putting a smile on their faces no matter how bad they feel. When I was leaving a hospital after visiting a young girl, the nurse said to me, "She's been having chemotherapy. Her hair fell out. But you're the first person who has been able to make her smile and laugh." That's the best feeling in the world. It's a better feeling than the rush of 80,000 fans cheering for me after scoring a touchdown.

I get a kick out of spending quality time with people who are simply looking for conversation and camaraderie, whether it is kids in hospitals or seniors in senior centers. My first job was working as an assistant at a nursing home in Lynwood, California. I spent most of the time playing cards with five older women.

These days, my perfect world is a place where people care enough to take the time to stop by schools and talk to kids. I've always been active in the Boys & Girls Clubs of America and often visit the kids in Kansas City or in Huntington Beach. I'll stop by and play pool, play Ping-Pong, or shoot hoops.

"TOO MANY OF US ONLY TAKE. WE DON'T GIVE. THIS IS TRUE WITH ALL AMERICANS, BUT ESPECIALLY ATHLETES AND ENTERTAINERS, WHO ARE ABLE TO TAKE SO MUCH BUT RARELY GIVE ENOUGH. I TRIED TO GIVE BACK ON THE FOOTBALL FIELD BY PROVIDING AN OUTLET, A DIVERSION FROM LIFE FOR A FEW HOURS ON A SUNDAY AFTERNOON, BUT THAT ISN'T ENOUGH. FAME IS WHAT YOU HAVE TAKEN, CHARACTER IS WHAT YOU GIVE. I WANTED TO HAVE CHARACTER BECAUSE FOOTBALL ALREADY GAVE ME FAME.

—Walter Payton, Former Running Back for the Chicago Bears

Living generously simply means that I have a chance to put positive energy, love, and compassion out into the universe. I believe that the only way to get anything out of life is to do good things for others and to be self-sacrificing. It sounds so simple, and yet becoming a caring person seems to be a struggle for many people in the world today.

7. HAVE FUN!

This is just as important as all the rest! You have to make sure you have fun in life. Have a positive attitude. Be grateful for the things you have. Enjoy your family and friends.

What's funny about my second season with the Chiefs (my sophomore year) is that I failed, despite working very hard to succeed. I didn't go out very much with my friends. I spent extra time in the weight room. I didn't drink or socialize. It sounds good in theory, but I ended up having the worst season of my entire career.

The harsh truth is that I was taking myself too seriously. I see a lot of athletes make this same mistake. You have to relax and be yourself. I was doing things that were out of character for me. I wasn't having fun, going out, and having social dinners with my friends. I would tell people I had to head home and go to sleep. I was taking creatine and other weight-gain products. I was 250 pounds and strong as an ox, but at the expense of speed and flexibility.

The problem, though, was more mental than physical. I needed to just relax and have a good time. I was putting too much pressure on myself. This was typical behavior of a young guy who could not focus. There's a tape from a game in my sophomore year that shows a ball being thrown to me, and sure enough I dropped it. Following the play, I was prone on the ground and hitting the ground as hard as I could with my fists, filled with frustration over dropping the ball. If I could go back and talk to that younger version of Tony, I'd tell him, "Get the hell off the ground! What are you doing? Don't be an idiot. Move on to the next play and don't worry about what happened."

8. TAKE ACTION.

You may have the tools you need and a plan in front of you, but unless you take action, change will never happen. It's time to get out of the huddle and make that play. Go for it!

I learned a big lesson about this during, again, my sophomore year in the NFL. As you can tell, I learned more in that year than any other season of my career. It was a growth spurt in my development in just one season. (And the lessons really worked, because I've been to the Pro Bowl every season since that second season.) I was getting the physical side of the game. In my sophomore year, I started *actively* taking part in my growth as an athlete from the mental side of the equation.

I encourage every athlete at every level to read about great athletes and what they do and how you can incorporate that into what you do and what makes sense for you. Everyone works differently. There's a formula for success to follow that builds on confidence and visualization and proper nutrition. But you will discover things that work better for you, depending on your own unique growth experience.

Developing a mindset is a personal experience. You can get a coach to tell you "this is how it's done," but until you actively take it upon yourself and start studying, you won't figure out what aspect of the mindset will work for your individual needs. Building the right mentality for success is like going to school or learning how to play a sport. You have to train your mind how to react and how to act.

For instance, I will run an out pattern on the field every day in practice. By practicing the drill, I will know how many steps it takes to get to 10 yards, and how to fake the defender in, and then I have to swim (shed) him off if he's going to grab me, and I have to cut out of the break at full speed. I do this every day in practice. I do it mentally, too, by quieting my mind. You have to learn to live in the present so that you can avoid thinking about the play coming up. You have to learn how not to let the crowd get into your head. You have to learn this stuff from experience. There's a reason why people go to church every week and study that same book—they want that book to become a part of them. That type of constant repetition is essential if you want to achieve greatness.

TAKING THIS MESSAGE TO THE WORLD

The All-Pro Diet for nutrition, fitness, and mental conditioning was created to help you fulfill all of your goals and aspirations to become a healthier person and improve your performance whether you are an athlete or not. The last piece of the puzzle is taking *your* newfound sense of physical well-being and using it to help other people.

I wrote this book to share my vision for a healthier world. You have every reason to be proud that you put the time and effort into working hard to be your absolute best.

Good for you. Your hard work will pay off!

APPENDIX A

Know the Difference Between a Nutritionist and a Registered Dietitian

If you want any individualized advice about your diet, make sure you are getting it from the right person. If you had a legal question, you probably would ask a lawyer, just as you would likely ask a doctor if you had a medical question. You should take the same expert-seeking approach with your nutritional health. A few good questions to ask to determine if the person is qualified are:

- What are his credentials?
- How many years has she been giving nutrition advice?
- Does he have experience working with athletes or active people?
- Does she require you to purchase any brand-name products as part of her services (that is, is she trying to sell you something)?

Nutrition advice should come from a registered dietitian. Unlike a nutritionist, who does not require any special qualifications, there are specific prerequisites for becoming an RD. These are:

- Complete a minimum 4-year bachelor of science degree in dietetics (nutrition) or a related science.
- Within the degree program, complete additional coursework required by the American Dietetic Association to be eligible for an internship.
- Complete a dietetic internship program (which averages 1 year in length).
- Pass the national registration exam created by the American Dietetic Association.
- Maintain 75 units of continuing education every 5 years to stay current.

To find a board-certified specialist in sports dietetics (CSSD), the highest professional sports nutrition credential in the United States, visit www.scandpg.org.

APPENDIX B

Statements from Authorities

WHAT IT TAKES

Jeff Hurd, my former strength coach with the Kansas City Chiefs, is now the strength and conditioning coach for the Chargers. Here are some of his observations about the work we did together when he was with the Chiefs as well as his advice on training and conditioning.

Tony is a consummate pro; he takes his job very seriously. And that mindset of professionalism and determination means he will work as hard as necessary to be the best tight end in pro football. That's why he works so hard in the weight room and before, during, and after practice. He's constantly doing extra drills on his routes and his footwork. He is very meticulous and disciplined on and off the football field. He never missed a single workout in all the time I was the Kansas City Chiefs' strength and conditioning coach. You can't say that about a lot of players. The difference with Tony is that he made the most of every single workout session for the 9 years we were together in Kansas City.

Tony is a fierce competitor. He really challenged himself every time he came into the weight room. He could be his own worst enemy because his expectations for his performance were very high. He has always been very team-oriented. I've heard him say on many occasions that he'd trade any personal achievement or stat for a win. But his mentality has always been that he has to be at his personal best for the Chiefs to have the best opportunity to win.

When he first started his pro career, there were questions about whether Tony could block at the NFL level. Whatever he thought his weakness was, in the weight room or on the football field, then that's what he paid the most attention to in his training. That's what makes him great. It's easy to work at what you are good at in your career. The trick is to have the guts to admit you need to make improvements and then focus on making those improvements through sweat, hard work, and endless repetition.

Like Tony, I believe that you get strong from the middle out, and so your core (lower back, glutes, abdominals, overall torso) has to be extremely strong. You play the game of football with your legs and your shoulders—if you can keep those areas strong, flexible, and powerful, you will be able to play at a very high level.

One of the keys to Tony's success was that he made the commitment to doing power cleans, squats, and lunges—the big three movements for football. He had injured his back in the weight room and that made him a little leery of doing the heavy core movements. Once he made a renewed commitment to those core lifts, his physical transformation was amazing! He became so incredibly strong. You have to credit his parents and the good Lord for his incredible athleticism. But his strength, power, change of direction, and balance are based on his hard work in the weight room. Everything starts with the legs and the core. Once those areas are strong, the power generates out to your hands, and that is what you need for blocking top-level NFL players.

Power cleans and squats are the two most important lifts. Nowadays everyone keeps inventing all these fancy new core workouts. That's fine. But the core movements that have stood the test of time are what you need to base your program upon.

The goal is to do squats and power cleans so that you don't get pushed around on the field, and they are also very important for balance and injury prevention. Now, I'm not saying that machines don't have a place in your workout, as they isolate certain muscle groups. The limitation of a machine is that it doesn't require any balance. When you're on the football field, though, your opponent does not stand still for you. He's moving. Not only do you have to develop strength, but you have to be able to balance and control him—and that's exactly what you do during free weight lifts.

There's more than one way to build strength. Just as some teams run the football and others pass the football, the ultimate objective is to figure out what you need to be successful, and there are many ways to do this. Tony believes, and it's what I teach, that all weight-training moves have to carry over to the football field.

When I was the Chiefs' strength coach, I always wished that Tony stayed in Kansas City and worked out with the team during the off-season. But I never worried about him. He always showed up in great shape. He communicated with me over the course of the off-season. He took the workout book home with him during the off-season. And he always arrived at training camp in superb physical condition and ready to play football, ready to go. Tony always backed up what he said he would do.

But the main reason I wanted Tony in Kansas City year-round was because of his positive influence on our younger players. When Tony would come back to Kansas City for on-the-field training sessions—and I want to make it clear that he would always come back whenever football practice was going on—the younger players were so impressed with his work ethic. He trains hard! He was always a step ahead of all the guys with his dedication to training.

As Tony has gotten older, his physical conditioning program has progressed and become even more of a priority, and it has paid off with a long and prosperous career. The guys who are in the NFL for a long time find a way to take care of their conditioning requirements. The game they play is not a normal activity—it's very violent, very taxing, and if you don't take care of your body, it won't last. Tony G.'s success is proof that hard work pays off.

A lot of younger players don't respect the history of training hard for football. Tony has always had tremendous respect for the hard work of the players who built the NFL, the guys who made the NFL what it has become. Tony has taken it upon himself to help the young guys appreciate the history of hard work in the NFL. He's a great role model and a great person, a leader.

A Vegan Diet for Professional Athletes: Is It Ideal?

Susan M. Kleiner, PhD, RD, FACN, CNS, FISSN, is the author of *Power Eating*, Third Edition (Human Kinetics, 2007) and *The Good Mood Diet* (Springboard Press, 2007), and the owner and president of High Performance Nutrition, LLC, in Mercer Island, Washington. Dr. Kleiner has also served as a sports nutrition consultant for the Seattle Seahawks and the Cleveland Browns.

There are so many good things about a plant-based diet: nutrients, fibers, and phytochemicals that enhance mental and physical performance and health. But a vegan diet for a pro athlete is a very hard strategy to follow practically, and it may result in less than optimal nutrition.

An athlete needs many calories, with carbs, protein, and fat allowing for that high-calorie intake. While the amount of fiber in a vegan diet is great for the average individual, an athlete may become so full from beans and whole grains that he can't eat enough food to get optimal levels of carbs, proteins, and fats. Athletes need to be very active for most of the day, and that feeling of fullness can also have a negative impact on performance and make them unable to run very fast. And while soy and tofu are excellent proteins containing the full spectrum of essential amino acids, some scientific findings show that men should not use soy as their sole source of protein. Additionally, that choice would create a narrow diet, from which no one would benefit, athlete or otherwise.

Another practical point is that, when traveling, it is difficult for a pro athlete to find the kinds of proteins needed to fulfill his daily protein needs. The convenience and availability of animal proteins that are lean or fat-free become virtually an essential part of an athlete's diet plan. This is why whey protein isolate is such a popular supplement.

Lastly, any diet devoid of fish must be supplemented with EPA (eicosapentaenoic acid) and DHA (docosahexaenoic acid), both omega-3 fatty acids. These can come from algae supplements, which are not yet widely available. Marine oils are absolutely essential for the health of the brain, cardiovascular system, and central nervous system.

The findings from the last decade of research into optimal protein consumption for enhancing strength and power have been quite clear. When calorie needs are met, protein needs range from 0.73 to 0.91 gram per pound of body weight per day, depending on the training cycle of the athlete. The goal of an athlete's diet is to maximize and optimize performance. They are not looking for adequate protein and adequate performance; they are trying to consistently achieve a personal record and then exceed that record again. Optimizing dietary intakes of proteins, fats, and carbohydrates will make a huge contribution to that goal.

RESOURCE GUIDE

AeroGrow: AeroGarden

Grow your own herbs, greens, and other foods inside your home. The AeroGarden is the first indoor smart garden.

www.aerogrow.com
customerservice@aerogrow.com
T: 800-476-9669

Almond Board of California

Additional recipes and information about almonds.

www.almondsarein.com
staff@almondboard.com
T: 209-549-8262

California Walnut Commission

Additional recipes and information about walnuts.

www.walnuts.org
wmbcwc@walnuts.org
T: 916-932-7070

CLIF Nectar Energy Bars

Made with five or fewer 100% organic ingredients. Every bar contains two servings of fruit.

www.clifbar.com
T: 800-254-3227

Hass Avocado Board

Your source for additional avocado recipes and nutritional information.

www.avocadocentral.com

LÄRABAR Energy Bars

Delicious bars made with unsweetened fruits, nuts, and spices with no more than six ingredients in each bar. Unprocessed. Raw. No added sugar. Non-GMO. No soy. Vegan. Dairy-free. Gluten-free. Kosher.

www.larabar.com
info@larabar.com
T: 800-543-2147

National Honey Board

Your source for additional recipes and nutritional information about honey.

www.honey.com
T: 303-776-2337

PranaBar Energy Bars

Organic energy bars. No gluten. Vegan. No soy. Dairy-free.

www.pranabars.com
T: 800-440-6476

PURE Bar Energy Bars

Delicious organic raw energy bars. No gluten. Vegan. No soy. No refined sugar.

www.thepurebar.com
T: 888-568-PURE

Raw Revolution Organic Live Food Bars

Delicious organic raw energy bars. No gluten. Vegan. No soy. No refined sugar.

www.rawindulgence.com
info@rawindulgence.com
T: 866-498-4671

Sambazon Organic Açaí

Sambazon has the best-tasting açaí products, hands down.

www.sambazon.com
info@sambazon.com
T: 877-726-2296

Tony Gonzalez All-Pro

High-quality 100% plant-based protein powder as well as a 100 percent whey protein powder using only the highest quality ingredients from grass-fed cows. Available in most health food stores and online.

www.tonygonzalezallpro.com

Vita-Mix

High-performance blender that makes eating whole foods easier.

www.vita-mix.com
T: 800-848-2649

YouBar Customized Nutrition Bars

Create your very own energy bar with your favorite ingredients!

www.youbars.com
support@youbars.com
T: 866-682-2771

Zing Nutrition Bars

Energy bars made with natural ingredients and a good combination of carbohydrates, protein, and fat.

www.zingbars.com
T: 206-362-3989

INDEX

Boldface page references indicate photographs. Underscored references indicate boxed text.

A

Açaí, 41, 69–70, 119, 124, 160
Accelerade, 167, 168–70
Acesulfame-K, 79, 119
Acupuncture, author's experience with, 5
Agave nectar, 59, 73–74, 159
ALA, 49, 51
Alcohol, 55–56, 78, 80, 81, 121–22
All-Pro Diet
　author's old diet compared to, 35
　benefits
　　for author, 24–26
　　for you, 26–28, 28
　evolution of, 19–20
　food lists, 92–97
　meal plans
　　Phase II sample plans, 108–14
　　Phase I sample plans, 101–7
　nutrition principles, 38–60
　Phase I
　　action items, 77–79
　　meal plans, 101–7
　　moving to Phase II, 79–80
　Phase II
　　action items, 80–81
　　meal plans, 108–14
　switching to, 32–36, 60
Almond oil, 76, 146, 148–49, 155
Almonds, 142, 144
Alpha-linolenic acid (ALA), 49, 51
Alzheimer's disease, decrease risk with omega-3 fats, 49
Anabolic hormones, 171
Antinutrients, 70

Antioxidants
　in berries, 69–70
　in fruit juices, 119
　in fruits, 42
　in grapeseed extract, 70
　in spinach, 63
Apples, 143
Apricots, dried, 139
Artificial ingredients, in foods, 45–46, 81
Artificial sweeteners, 73–74, 79, 119, 121
Asparagus, 155
Aspartame, 73, 79, 119
Athleticism, 198
Attack plan. See Eight-point plan of attack
Attention deficit disorder, decrease risk with omega-3 fats, 49
Avocados, 157

B

Balance, importance of, 197
Balsamic vinegar, 146, 158
Banana
　Banana Oatmeal Protein Pancakes, 134
　Black Bean Burgers, 150
　freezing for smoothies, 126
　in smoothies, 126, 128, 130, 132–33
Beans
　list of recommended for All-Pro Diet, 94
　protein content, 65

Beans *(cont.)*
   recipes
      Black Bean Burgers, 150
      Black Bean Soup, 137
      Black Beans with Quinoa, 151
      Chicken Chili with White Beans,
        148
      Kamut Salad, 144
      Lentil and Brown Rice Salad,
        139
      Lentil Soup with Apricots, 139
      Napa Cabbage White Bean Soup,
        138
Beef
   grass-fed, 23, 31–32
   grass-finished, 32, 51, 78, 87
Bell's palsy, 5
Bench press, 198–99
Bent-over lateral raise, 194, **194**
Berries
   Berry Crumble, 159
   nutrients in, <u>92</u>
   in smoothies, 124–25, 127–28
Beverages
   calories in, 118–22
   list of recommended for All-Pro Diet,
     95–96
Bipolar disorder, decrease risk with
     omega-3 fats, 49
Blood glucose test, fasting, 14
Blood pressure, high, 13, <u>14</u>, 15, 48
Blueberries, 69, 124
Bok choy, 152
Bounders, 196, **196**
Boys & Girls Clubs of America, 214
Bread, white, 52, 77
Breakfast
   cereals, 85
   importance of healthy, 58–59
   meal plan suggestions, 101–14
   recipes
      Banana Oatmeal Protein Pancakes,
        134
      Vegetable Scramble, 135
Broccoli, <u>93</u>
Brown rice, 52, 77, 140
Butter, nondairy, 59

C

Cabbage
   Napa Cabbage White Bean Soup, 138
Caffeine, 44
Calcium
   daily requirement, 31
   in dairy products, 29–31
   nondairy sources of, 31
   supplement, 31
Calories
   in alcohol, 55–56, 121
   burned by Wii Sport games, <u>175</u>
   counting, 61, 99
   in drinks, 54–56, 118–22
   empty, 21
   in teaspoon of sugar, 57, 73
   tips for increasing intake, <u>172</u>
Cancer
   decreased risk with
     broccoli, <u>93</u>
     fiber, 74, 75
   in former NFL players, 13
   increased risk with
     phytoestrogens, 71
     red meat, 31
Carbohydrates
   All-Pro Diet recommendations, 72
   avoiding added sugars, 57, 72
   calculating recovery needs, 168–69
   cravings, 72, 73
   low-carb diet, disadvantages of,
     72
   refined, 52, 72
   sources of, 72
   spotting hidden sugars in food labels,
     73
Cashews, 152
Cereals, 85, 93
Cheese
   Gorgonzola, 141
   saturated fat in, 30, 44
Cherries, 124, 144, 160, 169
Cherry juice, 119
Chicken
   Chicken Chili with White Beans,
     148
   Chicken Curry Salad, 142

Children
    healthy nutrition for, 82–83
    obesity, 12
Cholesterol
    effect of trans fats on, 44–45
    lowering with fiber diet, 74, 75
    testing, 14
CLA, 32
CLIF Nectar energy bar, 66, 163
Coconut
    Banana Coconut Smoothie, 132
    milk, 126
    nectar, 124, 129
    oil, 76, 147, 159
Coffee, 44, 55
Cognitive function impairment,
        decrease risk with omega-3 fats,
        48–49
Community Supported Agriculture
        (CSA), 24, 90
Condiments, 96
Conjugated linoleic acid (CLA), 32
Constipation, preventing with high-fiber
        diet, 74, 75
Cookies, 57, 59, 87
Cooking
    enjoyment of, 75
    supplies, 76
Cooking oils, 76
Corn syrup, high-fructose, 54, 57, 72–73,
        167
Coronary disease, 13, 14, 44–45
Cortisol, 167
Cranberries, 141, 160
Cravings, carbohydrates, 72, 73
Creatine, 70, 215
Crunches, 180–81, **180–81**
Crystal Light, 79, 119, 121
CSA, 24, 90

D

Dairy products
    controlling in diet, 28–31
    list of recommended for All-Pro Diet,
        94
    organic, 87, 88

osteoporosis and, 29, 30
    protein content, 65
Dehydration, 43, 164–65, 167
Depression, role of omega-3 fats in
        prevention of, 49
Dessert recipes
    Açaí Quinoa Dessert, 160
    Berry Crumble, 159
DHA, 49, 51
Diabetes
    in children, 82
    complications of, 15
    increase in prevalence of, 8, 12
    increase risk with
        fruit drinks, 55
        obesity, 8, 12–13
    metabolic syndrome (prediabetes),
        13–16, 55
Diet plan, starting new, 25
Diet soda, 54
Digestive problems, dairy-product
        associated, 29
Dinners, meal plan suggestion for,
        101–14
Discipline, importance of, 199–200
Diverticular disease, 74–75
Docosahexaenoic acid (DHA), 49, 51
Dumbbell bench press, 189, **189**
Dumbbell curl, 195, **195**
Dumbbell lateral raise, 193, **193**

E

Eating
    frequency of, 41
    late-night, avoiding, 59
    for performance
        after exercise, 168–71
        before exercise, 163–64, 164
        during exercise, 166–68
    portion control, 52–53, 115
    speed of, 53–54, 78, 80
    stopping when satisfied, 53–54,
        78
    weekend, 56
Eating habits, 23
Eating out, 115–17

Eggs
  omega-3 fats in, 51
  protein content, 64
  Vegetable Scramble, 135
Eicosapentaenoic acid (EPA), 49, 51
Eight-point plan of attack, 203–17
  goals, setting, 208–9
  good people, surrounding yourself
    with, 206
  having fun, 215–16
  living generously, 213–15
  personal relationships, building,
    207–8
  reading, 204–6
  taking action, 216–17
  working hard, 210–13
Endurance, improving with All-Pro Diet,
  4
Energy bar, 66, 118, 163–64, 167
EPA, 49, 51
Equal, 73, 79
Exercise
  bench press, 198–99
  bent-over lateral raise, 194, **194**
  bounders, 196, **196**
  dumbbell bench press, 189, **189**
  dumbbell curl, 195, **195**
  dumbbell lateral raise, 193, **193**
  jump rope, 179, **179**
  leg curl, 191, **191**
  lunge, 187, **187**
  medicine ball throw, 183, **183**
  power clean, 175–76, 185, **185**
  pullup, 178, 192, **192**
  RDLs, 188, **188**
  shoulder shrug, 190, **190**
  side crunch, 181, **181**
  sport-specific, 175–76
  squat, 176, 177–78, 186, **186**
  straight crunch, 180, **180**
  yugo, 182, **182**

F

Facial paralysis, 5
Farmers' market, 23, 78, 80, <u>83</u>, 86–87
Fast food, 53, 58, 79, <u>83</u>

Fats
  list of recommended for All-Pro Diet,
    95
  omega-3, 47–51, <u>96</u>
  omega-6, 48, 49
  polyunsaturated, 48
  saturated, 29, 30, 31, 44, 51, 67
  trans, 44–45
Fiber, 47, <u>74</u>, 74–75
Fish
  American Heart Association
    recommendations on, 51
  list of recommended for All-Pro Diet,
    95
  mercury in, 50–51
  omega-3 fats in, 49–51
  as protein source, 40, 64
  recipes
    Cilantro Grilled Salmon, 145
    Fish Tacos, 149
    Lemon Honey Mahi Mahi, 146
Fish oil supplements, 49, 51, 78
Flavonoids, <u>86</u>
Flaxseed/flaxseed oil, 49, 51, 68–70, 128
Flour, refined, 52, 77, 79
Fluids
  calculating your basic requirement, 43,
    165
  calories from, 54–56, 118–22
  dehydration, 43, 164–65, <u>167</u>
  NATA fluid replacement guidelines,
    <u>165</u>
  sports drinks during workouts, 166–67
  water bottle use for tracking intake,
    <u>166</u>
Focus, 4, 206, 209, 215
Food labels, spotting hidden sugars in, 73
Food log, 62
Foods
  artificial ingredients, 45–46, 81
  calcium sources, 31
  for children, <u>82–83</u>
  color, <u>92</u>
  convenience, 86
  to eliminate from diet, 78–79
  enjoying what we eat, 27–28, 32–33,
    47

fast, 53, 58, 79, <u>83</u>
fiber sources, <u>74</u>
immediate changes in diet, list for, 81
junk, 9, 71
list of worst and best, <u>18</u>
local, 23, <u>24</u>, 80, 84, 87, 90
omega-3 fat sources, 49–51
organic, 23, <u>24</u>, 80, 85, 87–88
pesticides in, 23, <u>24</u>, 71, 87–90
processed, 45–47, 71, 78, 80, 83–84
protein sources, 64–66
Slow Food movement, 90–91
thermic effect of food, 63
unwanted list, 97–98
vitamin D sources, <u>30</u>
Food shopping
cost savings, 84–86
frequency of trips, 78
plan of action, 82–84
Free radicals, 69
Fries, sweet potato, 156
Fruit juice, 55, 119, 120
Fruits
antioxidants in, 42
benefits in diet, 42–43
canned, 79
list of recommended for All-Pro Diet,
92
natural sugars, 73
organic, 87–88
recommended daily intake, 43, 72
Fun, 215–16

G

Gatorade, 167
GatorLytes, 166
Gazpacho, 136
Genes, effect of lifestyle choices on, <u>46</u>
Glycogen, replenishing stores of, <u>170</u>,
171
Gnu energy bar, 118, 163
Goals, setting, 208–9
Goitrogens, in soy, 71
Goji berries, 70
Good people, surrounding yourself with,
206

Grains
list of recommended for All-Pro Diet,
93
protein content, 65
whole, 40–41, 52, <u>83</u>
Granola, 58
Grape juice, 119
Grapes, <u>96</u>, 142, 143
Grapeseed oil/extract, 70, 142–43
Green tea, <u>86</u>
Grocery shopping. *See* Food shopping
Growth hormone, 171
Guacamole, 157

H

HDL, 14
Health problems, of NFL players,
12–13
Health profile, <u>25</u>
Health scares, of author, 5–7
Heart disease
antiaging effects of resveratrol, <u>96</u>
decreased risk with
fiber, 74
green tea, <u>86</u>
moderate alcohol consumption, <u>80</u>
omega-3 fats, 48, 51
increased risk with
diabetes, 15
obesity, 13
saturated and trans fats, 44–45
Hemagglutinin, in soy, 71
Hemp milk, <u>88</u>, 124–35
Hemp protein powder, 70
Herbs, 96
High-density lipoprotein (HDL), 14
High-fructose corn syrup, 54, 57, 72–73,
167
Holtz, Lou, 203, 206, 211
Honey, 73, 134, 146
Hormones, anabolic, 171
Hydration, 43–44, 164–65, <u>165</u>
Hydrogenation, 44, 45, 79
Hypertension (high blood pressure), 13,
<u>14</u>, 15, 48
Hyponatremia, 166

I

Ice cream, rice, 33
Insulin, 14, 171
Insulin-like growth factor-1 (IGF-1), 171

J

Joint health, improvement with omega-3
    fats, 48
Jordan, Michael, 210–11
Juice, fruit, 55, 119, 120
Jump rope, 179, **179**
Junk food, 9, 71

K

Kamut, 144

L

Lactase, 29
Lactose intolerance, 29
LÄRABAR energy bar, 66, 118, 163
LDL, 44
Lean protein, 40–41, <u>67</u>
Leg curl, 191, **191**
Leg press, 177–78
Legumes, 65, 94
Lentils
    Lentil and Brown Rice Salad, 139
    Lentil Soup with Apricots, 139
Life expectancy, 85, <u>91</u>
Lifestyle choices, effect on genes, <u>46</u>
Liquid nutrition
    after exercise, 169–70
    digestibility, 169
Living generously, 213–15
Log, food, 62
Lombardi, Vince, 205–6, 210
Low-density lipoprotein (LDL), 44
Lunch, meal plan suggestions for, 101–14
Lunge, 187, **187**

M

Macadamia nut oil, 76, 137–39, 147, 151,
    154, 156

Macadamia nuts, 58
Machines, 178
Mahi mahi, 146
Main dish recipes
    Black Bean Burgers, 150
    Chicken Chili with White Beans, 148
    Cilantro Grilled Salmon, 145
    Fish Tacos, 149
    Lemon Honey Mahi Mahi, 146
    Whole Wheat Linguine with Shrimp,
        147
Mango, 129
Maple syrup, 59
Meal plans
    Phase II sample plans, 108–14
        Day 1, 108
        Day 2, 109
        Day 3, 110
        Day 4, 111
        Day 5, 112
        Day 6, 113
        Day 7, 114
    Phase I sample plans, 101–7
        Day 1, 101
        Day 2, 102
        Day 3, 103
        Day 4, 104
        Day 5, 105
        Day 6, 106
        Day 7, 107
    steps to planning, 100
Meals
    number per day, 41–42
    sample day, 42
    skipping, 56–57
Meat
    expense of, 84
    grass-finished/grass-fed beef, 23,
        31–32, 51, 78, 87
    highly processed, eliminating, 79
    limiting consumption of red, 78
    list of recommended for All-Pro Diet,
        95
    poultry, free-range, 23, 87, 115
    protein content, 64
    saturated fat in red meat, 31
Medicine ball, 175

Medicine ball throw, 183, **183**
Memory loss, decrease risk with omega-3
    fats, 48
Mercury
    dangers of, <u>50</u>
    in fish, 50–51
Metabolic syndrome, 13–16, 55
Metabolism
    boost from protein, 63, <u>67</u>
    impact of missing meal on, 56
    thermic effect of food, 63
Milk
    controlling in diet, 29–31
    hemp, <u>88</u>, 124–35
    saturated fat in, 44
Mindset for success, 216
Miso, 71, 94
Multivitamin, 68–69, 78
Muscle building/growth
    optimizing with recovery nutrition,
        <u>170</u>, 171
    protein and, 62, 64, 66–67
    tips for natural, <u>172</u>
Muscle soreness, reducing, 168, <u>170</u>

N

Natto, 71, 95
NFL
    health problems of players, 12–13
    off-season workout programs, 174, 199
    team nutritionist, goals of, <u>6</u>
Nut butters, 94, 131
NutraSweet, 73, 79
Nutrient timing, 67
Nutrition, All-Pro Diet principles of,
    38–60
Nutritionist
    author's experience with Mitzi Dulan,
        7–12
    goals of NFL team, <u>6</u>
    role of sports nutritionists, <u>10</u>
Nuts
    list of recommended for All-Pro Diet,
        94
    protein content, 65
    walnuts, 49, 51, 141, 143

O

Oatmeal, 58, 134
Oats, rolled, 127, 134, 159
Obesity
    in America, 7, 12
    childhood, 12, <u>82</u>
    family history, 12
    health issues associated with
        diabetes, 8, 12–13
        heart disease, 12
        premature death, 12
        preventable, 15–16
    in NFL players, 12–13
    severe, 12
Oils
    hydrogenated, 44, 45, 79
    list of recommended for All-Pro Diet,
        95
Okinawa, longevity of population, 85,
    <u>91</u>
Olive oil, 76, 144
Omega-3 fats, 47–51, <u>96</u>
Omega-6 fats, 48, 49
Orange juice, 119
Organic foods, 23, <u>24</u>, 80, 85, 87–88
Osteoporosis, <u>29</u>, 30
Overweight individuals, in America, 12,
    <u>82</u>

P

Pain, 19, 25
Pancakes, 134
Partially hydrogenated vegetable oil, 45
Peaches, 129
Peanut butter, 79
Personal relationships, building, 207–8
Pesticides, 23, <u>24</u>, 71, 87–90
Phenolic compounds, 119
Phytate, in soy, 70–71
Phytoestrogens, in soy, 71
Phytonutrients, 42, 47, <u>63</u>, <u>92</u>
Plant-based foods
    incorporating into diet, 21, 23, 77, 80
    omega-3 fats in, 49
    protein sources, <u>67</u>, 68–70
Polyunsaturated fats (PUFAs), 48

Pop Warner football, author's experience
     with, 211–12
Portion control, 52–53, 115
Potassium loss, 166
Poultry, free-range, 23, 87, 115
Power clean, 175–76, 185, **185**
PranaBar energy bar, 66, 118
Preservatives, in food, 45–46, 79, 81
Processed foods, 45–47, 71, 78, 80,
     83–84
Prostate cancer, preventing, <u>93</u>
Protein
     benefits of, 62–63
     calculating recovery needs, 169
     calculating your own daily
          requirement, 64
     fast, 68
     higher needs of physically active
          people, 62–63
     lean, 40–41, <u>67</u>
     plant-based, <u>67</u>, 68–70
     RDA recommendation, 62
     sources, 31, 40, 60, 64–66
     timing consumption of, 67
Protein powders
     in Banana Oatmeal Protein Pancakes,
          134
     hemp, 70
     importance in diet, 67
     plant-based, 68–70
     in smoothie recipes, 124–25
     whey, 68
PUFAs, 48
Pullup, 178, 192, **192**
PURE Bar energy bar, 66, 118, 163

Q

Quinoa
     Açaí Quinoa Dessert, 160
     Black Beans with Quinoa, 151
     Quick Quinoa, 154
Quotations
     Bok, Edward, 212
     Cossman, E. Joseph, 210
     Dulan, Mitzi, 3
     Edison, Thomas, 174

Edwards, Herm, 173
Holmes, Sr., Oliver Wendell, 38
Holtz, Lou, 203, 211
Lincoln, Abraham, 163
Maxwell, John, 213
Mays, Willie, 94
Nicklaus, Jack, 12
Noll, Chuck, 77
Payton, Walter, 214
Peale, Norman Vincent, 61
Polan, Michael, 17
Richardson, Tony, 6
Riley, Pat, 99
Sills, Beverly, 34
Skolnik, Heidi, 6
Smith, May B., 210
Stoddard, Alexandra, 123
Truman, Harry S., 208
Trump, Donald, 198
von Goethe, Johann Wolfgang,
     176
Waitley, Denis, 21
Washington, Booker T., 206

R

Raw Revolution energy bar, 66, 118
RDA, 62
RDLs, 188, **188**
Reading, value of, 204–6
Recipes
     breakfast
          Banana Oatmeal Protein Pancakes,
               134
          Vegetable Scramble, 135
     desserts
          Açaí Quinoa Dessert, 160
          Berry Crumble, 159
     main dishes
          Black Bean Burgers, 150
          Chicken Chili with White Beans,
               148
          Cilantro Grilled Salmon, 145
          Fish Tacos, 149
          Lemon Honey Mahi Mahi, 146
          Whole Wheat Linguine with Shrimp,
               147

salads
   Chicken Curry Salad, 142
   Kamut Salad, 144
   Lentil and Brown Rice Salad, 140
   Spinach Salad, 141
   Waldorf Salad, 143
sides
   Baby Bok Choy with Cashews, 152
   Balsamic Vinaigrette, 158
   Black Beans with Quinoa, 151
   Easy Asparagus, 155
   Easy Steamed Spinach, 153
   Guacamole, 157
   Quick Quinoa, 154
   Sweet Potato Fries, 156
smoothies
   Banana Berry Smoothie, 128
   Banana Coconut Smoothie, 132
   Chocolate Banana Smoothie, 130
   Chocolate Nut Butter Smoothie,
     131
   Coconut Dream Smoothie, 126
   Mitzi's Berrylicious Smoothie, 125
   Oatmeal Berry Bliss Smoothie, 127
   Peach Mango Smoothie, 129
   Planet Earth Smoothie, 133
   Tony's Morning Power Smoothie,
     124
soups
   Black Bean Soup, 137
   Lentil Soup with Apricots, 139
   Napa Cabbage White Bean Soup,
     138
   Quick Gazpacho, 136
Recommended Dietary Allowances
   (RDA), 62
Recovery
  benefits of All-Pro Diet for, 4, 24–26
  drink recipes
   Banana Berry Smoothie, 128
   Banana Coconut Smoothie, 132
   Chocolate Banana Smoothie, 130
   Chocolate Nut Butter Smoothie,
     131
   Coconut Dream Smoothie, 126
   Mitzi's Berrylicious Smoothie, 125
   Oatmeal Berry Bliss Smoothie, 127

   Peach Mango Smoothie, 129
   Planet Earth Smoothie, 133
   Tony's Morning Power Smoothie,
     124
nutrition plan
   benefits, 168, 170
   carbohydrates, 168–69
   liquids vs. solid, 169–70
   protein, 169
Red meat
  limiting consumption of, 31, 78
  saturated fat in, 31
Red wine, 96
Refined carbohydrates, 52
Relationships, importance of, 207–8
Repetition, value of, 216–17
Restaurants, eating at, 115–17, 118
Resveratrol, 96
Rice, 52, 77, 140
Robbins, Tony, 26, 206
Role models, professional athletes as, 213

S

Saccharin, 73, 79
Salad recipes
   Chicken Curry Salad, 142
   Kamut Salad, 144
   Lentil and Brown Rice Salad, 140
   Spinach Salad, 141
   Waldorf Salad, 143
Salmon
   Cilantro Grilled Salmon, 145
Salt table, 166
Satiety, 62, 63
Saturated fats, 29, 30, 31, 44, 51, 67
Seafood
  list of recommended for All-Pro Diet,
    95
  Whole Wheat Linguine with Shrimp,
    147
Seeds
  list of recommended for All-Pro Diet,
    94
  protein content, 65
Seitan, 100
Self-confidence, building, 210, 212

Self-help books, 206
Sesame oil, 152
Shadow Buddy, 213–14
Shopping. *See* Food shopping
Shoulder shrug, 190, **190**
Shrimp, 147
Side crunch, 181, **181**
Sides
    Baby Bok Choy with Cashews, 152
    Balsamic Vinaigrette, 158
    Black Beans with Quinoa, 151
    Easy Asparagus, 155
    Easy Steamed Spinach, 153
    Guacamole, 157
    Quick Quinoa, 154
    Sweet Potato Fries, 156
Skin, improvement with All-Pro Diet,
    27
Slow Food movement, 90–91
Smoke point, of cooking oils, 76
Smoothies
    prior to exercising, 164
    recipes
        Banana Berry Smoothie, 128
        Banana Coconut Smoothie, 132
        Chocolate Banana Smoothie, 130
        Chocolate Nut Butter Smoothie,
            131
        Coconut Dream Smoothie, 126
        Mitzi's Berrylicious Smoothie, 125
        Oatmeal Berry Bliss Smoothie,
            127
        Peach Mango Smoothie, 129
        Planet Earth Smoothie, 133
        Tony's Morning Power Smoothie,
            124
    as recovery drink, 169–70
Snacks
    All-Pro Diet ideas for, 97
    before exercise, 163–64, <u>164</u>
    late-night, avoiding, 59
    meal plan suggestions, 101–14
    number per day, 41–42
    planning for, 86
    plant-based, 80
    for traveling, 115, 118
    during workout, 167

Soda, 54–55, 119, 121
Sodium
    hyponatremia, 166
    in sports drinks, 166
Sodium nitrate/nitrite, 79
Soup recipes
    Black Bean Soup, 137
    Lentil Soup with Apricots, 139
    Napa Cabbage White Bean Soup,
        138
    Quick Gazpacho, 136
Soy foods
    dangers associated with, 70–71, <u>71</u>
    fermented, 71, 94
    protein in, 65, 70
Sperm count, reduction from high-soy
    diet, <u>71</u>
Spices, 96
Spinach
    Easy Steamed Spinach, 153
    nutrients in, <u>63</u>
    in smoothies, <u>63</u>, 124–25, 133
    Spinach Salad, 141
    Whole Wheat Linguine with Shrimp,
        147
Splenda, 73, 79
Sports drinks
    calories in, 121
    during workouts, 166–67
Squat, 176, 177–78, 186, **186**
Stevia, 73, 74
Straight crunch, 180, **180**
Strawberries, 124, 159
Stroke, 13, 15, 44
Sucralose, 73, 79, 119
Sugars
    avoiding added, 57, 72–73
    high-fructose corn syrup, 54, 57,
        72–73, 167
    spotting hidden, in food labels, 73
    World Health Organization
        recommendation, 57
Sulforaphane, <u>93</u>
Sunett, 79
Supplements
    calcium, 31
    fish oil, 49, 51, 78

multivitamin, 68–69, 78
protein, 66, 67–70
Sweeteners
artificial, 73–74, 79, 119, 121
in diet soda, 54–55
on food label ingredient list, 73
high-fructose corn syrup, 54, 57,
72–73, 167
natural, 59, 73–74, 96
Sweet'N Low, 73, 79
Sweet potato, 156
Sweets, cravings for, 72, 73
Syndrome X, 13–16

T

Taco, fish, 149
Taking action, 216–17
Tea, green, 86
Team nutritionist, goals of, 6
Tempeh, 71, 94, 100
Testosterone, 171
Tetrahydrocannabinol (THC), 70
Thermic effect of food, 63
Timing, nutrient, 67
Tofu, 71, 95
Tony Gonzalez Foundation, 213–14
Trainers, 177
Trans fats, 44–45
Traveling, nutritional tips for, 115–18
Triglycerides, 14, 48
Tuna, mercury in, 50

U

Unwanted foods list, 97–98

V

VAP test, 14
Vegan diet, 17–19, 31, 40
Vegetable oil
hydrogenated, 44, 45, 79
omega-6 fats in, 48
Vegetables
benefits in diet, 42–43
canned, 79

list of recommended for All-Pro Diet,
92–93
organic, 87–88
recipes
Easy Asparagus, 155
Easy Steamed Spinach, 153
Sweet Potato Fries, 156
Vegetable Scramble, 135
recommended daily intake, 43, 72
Vertical auto profile (VAP) test, 14
Visualization, 176, 206
Vitamins
multivitamin, 68–69, 78
in spinach, 63
Vitamin D, 30
vitamin E, in grass-finished beef,
32

W

Waffles, 59
Walnuts, 49, 51, 141, 143
Warm-up exercises
jump rope, 179, **179**
side crunch, 181, **181**
straight crunch, 180, **180**
yugo, 182, **182**
Water
bottled, 85
calculating your basic requirement, 43,
165
dehydration, 43, 164–65, 167
NATA fluid replacement guidelines,
165
tracking intake using water bottle,
166
Water bottle, 166
Water purifiers, 85
Weekend eating, 56
Weight gain
encouraged in NFL, 13
tips for natural, 172
Weight loss
promotion by avoiding late-night
eating, 59
tips for armchair quarterback, 22
tips for permanent, 37

Weight training
  author's off-season regimen, 174–75
  discipline and hard work, importance
      of, 199–200
  exercises, 184–96, **185–96**
      bent-over lateral raise, 194, **194**
      bounders, 196, **196**
      dumbbell bench press, 189, **189**
      dumbbell curl, 195, **195**
      dumbbell lateral raise, 193, **193**
      leg curl, 191, **191**
      lunge, 187, **187**
      power clean, 185, **185**
      pullup, 192, **192**
      RDLs, 188, **188**
      shoulder shrug, 190, **190**
      squat, 186, **186**
  free weights vs. machines, 178
  quality vs. quantity, 198–99
  sport-specific exercises, 175–76
  warm-up exercises, 179–83, **179–83**
Wheat germ, 134
Whey protein
  in Accelerade, 169
  powder, 68
Whole grains
  in All-Pro Diet, 40–41
  for children, 83
  choosing over refined carbohydrates,
      52

Wii (Nintendo), 175
Wine, 96
Woods, Tiger, 210
Working hard, 210–13
Workout
  author's approach to, 197–200
  changing exercises in, 177–78
  eating/nutrition plan
      after exercise, 168–71
      during exercise, 166–68
      fluid intake, 164–65, 165, 166,
          167
      prior to exercise, 163–64, 164
  professional help with, 177
  schedule, 174–75, 197, 199
  visualization, 176
  warm-up exercises, 179–83,
      179–83
  weight-training exercises, 184–96,
      185–96

Y

YouBar energy bar, 66, 163
Yugo, 182, **182**

Z

Zing energy bar, 66, 118, 163